Positiv

Positively Smarter

Science and Strategies for Increasing Happiness, Achievement, and Well-Being

Marcus Conyers and Donna Wilson, PhD

WILEY Blackwell

This edition first published 2015
© 2015 John Wiley & Sons, Inc.

Registered Office
John Wiley & Sons Ltd, The Atrium, Southern Gate, Chichester, West Sussex, PO19 8SQ, UK

Editorial Offices
350 Main Street, Malden, MA 02148-5020, USA
9600 Garsington Road, Oxford, OX4 2DQ, UK
The Atrium, Southern Gate, Chichester, West Sussex, PO19 8SQ, UK

For details of our global editorial offices, for customer services, and for information about how to apply for permission to reuse the copyright material in this book please see our website at www.wiley.com/wiley-blackwell.

The right of Marcus Conyers and Donna Wilson to be identified as the authors of this work has been asserted in accordance with the UK Copyright, Designs and Patents Act 1988.

Library of Congress Cataloging-in-Publication Data

Conyers, Marcus, author.
    Positively smarter : science and strategies for increasing happiness, achievement, and well-being / Marcus Conyers and Donna Wilson.
        pages cm
    Includes bibliographical references and index.
    ISBN 978-1-118-92609-3 (cloth) – ISBN 978-1-118-92610-9 (pbk.)   1. Well-being.
2. Happiness.   3. Metacognition.   4. Neuroplasticity.   I. Wilson, Donna (Psychologist), author.   II. Title.
    BF575.H27+

                                                                                        2015006915

A catalogue record for this book is available from the British Library.

Cover image: active nerve cell illustration – Stock Image / © Eraxion

Set in 11/13.5pt Plantin by Aptara Inc., New Delhi, India
Printed and bound in Malaysia by Vivar Printing Sdn Bhd

1   2015

This book is dedicated to the graduates of the master's and educational specialist degree programs with majors in brain-based teaching and the graduates in the doctoral minor in brain-based leadership at Nova Southeastern University. Thank you for all you are doing to help students, families, colleagues, schools, and communities to become positively smarter.

Contents

Acknowledgments

We gratefully acknowledge the hundreds of educators who have earned their graduate degrees in brain-based teaching and then shared with us the positive results that they, their colleagues, and their students are achieving in classrooms across the country and around the world. It has been inspirational to hear how these teachers and administrators have applied what they have learned—not only professionally but also at home, in particular with their own children, and in their communities. Their stories truly inspire us.

We'd also like to acknowledge the tremendous impact of theorists Reuven Feuerstein and Robert Sternberg, whose seminal work has greatly informed our own. Also in these pages, we share what we have learned from Robert Sylwester, who has brought clarity to the field of education in connecting the implications of brain science to classroom practice and who worked with us on our Scholarships for Teachers in Action Research with the Florida Department of Education.

A big thank you goes out to our reviewers for taking time from their busy schedules to carefully read and comment on our manuscript: Lisa Holder Lohmann, EdD, Associate Professor of Education at the University of Central Oklahoma; Kelly D. Rose, EdD, library media specialist at The Out-of-Door Academy, Sarasota, Florida; and Carol Mikulka, MD, psychiatrist and founder of the Walden Community School, Winter Park, Florida. Additionally, we are enormously thankful for our teammates Mary Collington and Mary Buday, who keep everything running smoothly so we can pursue our passion to write. Our wonderful editor, Karen Bankston, always does the job well and makes sure we stay within our deadlines, despite our obsession with adding new research all along the way. Thank you, Lorraine Ortner-Blake, for creating the great illustrations that accompany this text. We had the privilege to work with Acquisitions Editor Jayne Fargnoli, Senior Project Editor Julia Kirk, and other knowledgeable and helpful staff at Wiley Blackwell; we also appreciate the care that Project Manager and Copy Editor Joanna Pyke took with our manuscript.

Finally, we are grateful to have had the opportunity to work with one another in developing this book. It was a rewarding journey, giving us the opportunity to delve deeper into the practical applications of our work. We are pleased that we can share the implications of this work that has so greatly informed and enriched our lives. We have loved living the process described in this book.

Introduction
Redefining Potential as Our Neurocognitive Capacity to Get Better at (Almost) Anything

"The brain is a complex biological organ of great computational capability that constructs our sensory experiences, regulates our thoughts and emotions, and controls our actions."

—Eric Kandel, Nobel laureate[1]

The classic documentary *Private Universe*, produced by the Harvard-Smithsonian Center for Astrophysics, explores challenges in science education. In its opening scene, randomly selected graduates and faculty at a Harvard commencement are asked to explain why it is warm in the summer and cold in the winter. These bright young people who have had the advantage of the most sought-after education in the world happily list the science courses they took in high school and college and then embark on their descriptions of what causes the seasons. Most come down to a common conceptualization: The Earth's orbit around the sun is elliptical; when it passes nearest the sun, we have summer, and at the farthest reaches of its oval-shaped path, we dig out our winter coats and snow shovels. These Harvard graduates and several of their professors are well spoken and

Positively Smarter: Science and Strategies for Increasing Happiness, Achievement, and Well-Being, First Edition. Marcus Conyers and Donna Wilson.
© 2015 John Wiley & Sons, Inc. Published 2015 by John Wiley & Sons, Inc.

enthusiastic, and their astronomical interpretations are convincing, clearly explained, and—for 21 of the 23 people interviewed—just plain wrong.[2]

In much the same way, each of us relies on personal theories operating in our own "private universe," and these theories have a profound impact on how we think and feel and what we achieve in our lives. One of the most influential theories is how we perceive our potential to succeed in school, in work, and in life. What sets high achievers apart from others? What stands between us and our aims of finding happiness, excelling in educational and career pursuits, and achieving our personal goals?

One prevalent conception holds that people's potential for achieving these aims is determined by the pre-established portion of innate talent, inherited intelligence, and deep-seated predilection toward optimism or pessimism that determines the level of their progress and outlook on life. A big portion leads to big success, and a smaller portion limits the ability to move ahead. This conception holds that innate talent is obvious in how easily some people do well in school and excel in their chosen fields. The necessity to work hard indicates a lack of potential. Intelligence is fixed, and IQ scores predict with eerie certainty how well people will do in life.

This view of potential is quite common. In their book *Teaching for Wisdom, Intelligence, Creativity, and Success*, authors Robert Sternberg, Linda Jarvin, and Elena Grigorenko note that single-faceted views of general intelligence, such as one called the "*g*-factor theory," are based on beliefs that intelligence, ability, and outlook are fixed from birth by genetic endowment. "In other words, according to this theory, you are born with a certain amount of smarts and the type of schooling you receive won't change it that much."[3]

Writing about widely held perceptions of success, Heidi Grant Halvorson contends that culture has a powerful influence on how we think about achievement. Western societies tend to equate accomplishment with innate abilities and label people as *geniuses* and *prodigies* in a way that signals that their successes are rare and out of the reach of the rest of us "non-geniuses." Americans, especially, "celebrate people who we believe have special abilities and tend to see those who work hard to succeed as less innately capable."[4] Along the same lines, Carol Dweck has written extensively about the impact of a "fixed mindset," or the belief that intelligence and ability are largely unchangeable.[5] A group of British educational researchers sums up this perspective:

> It is widely believed that the explanation for the differences between individuals is that the likelihood of people becoming unusually competent in certain fields of accomplishment depends upon the presence or absence of attributes that have an inborn biological component, and are variously labeled "gifts" or "talents" or, less often, "natural aptitudes." It is thought that a young person is unlikely to become an exceptionally good musician, for example, unless he or she is among the minority of individuals who are, innately, musically "talented" or "gifted."[6]

K. Anders Ericsson, an eminent researcher on developing expert performance through what he describes as "deliberate practice," highlights similar findings about what many people believe about innate talent and performance. In an article in the journal *American Psychologist*, Ericsson and coauthor Neil Charness note that most people view the achievements of top performers in a variety of fields as so exceptional that this level of attainment must be attributed to unique inherent "gifts."[7]

These cultural beliefs are absorbed by children as they grow and may influence their level of motivation, attitudes about their abilities, and, ultimately, academic outcomes. In fact, this *g*-factor theory, this fixed mindset, this "secret" of success—call it what you will—influences the "private universe" of many children and adults and thus their optimism about their future and performance in school, in work, and in life. If you believe that achievement results from innate ability and if you have no evidence that you are gifted or talented, why try?

Appreciating Brain Plasticity: The Key to Redefining Potential

We advocate for a quite different perspective on the potential of all people to lead happier and healthier lives and to achieve their personal and career goals. This view rests on an understanding that the human brain has tremendous capacity to change and improve in response to experience. As a result, virtually all people have the capacity to learn, to grow, and to improve at whatever skills they choose through a positive outlook and the use of effective strategies, persistent effort, and deliberate practice. While innate ability may be part of the puzzle, we submit that conscious, deliberate practice, the development of new skills, optimism, and resilience are what really separate successful people from those who do not achieve their aims. This conception of potential to lead a happier, healthier, and more fulfilling life is supported by a wide range of research explored in this book about the power of the brain to become smarter, in terms of increased skills in solving problems, applying creativity, and learning new things throughout the life span; the body to become healthier and stronger; and the spirit to become more optimistic.

We define *potential* as the neurocognitive capacity for acquiring the knowledge, skills, and attitudes to achieve a higher level of performance in any domain. In other words, potential represents the power for getting better at whatever you set as your goals by rewiring your brain and body with new outlooks, knowledge, skills, and abilities. The foundations of human potential are built permanently into the brain's readiness for learning from infancy throughout one's life and in the ability of the brain and body to continually adapt to new challenges and learning.

The Path to Positively Smarter

The expression *positively smarter* captures the essence of increasing well-being across three interconnected domains of happiness,

4

achievement, and wellness. In this book we will explore research and strategies to:

1. **Increase our positivity, optimism, and happiness** (also referred to as *subjective well-being*). Through the effective use of key strategies to change our attitudes and outlook, we can become happier and more optimistic more of the time. Scientists have pinpointed areas of the brain that are more active when people are optimistic, have a positive outlook, and exhibit resilience.[8] Over the long term, these and other elements of emotional style can be improved by the application of practical strategies. These advances in knowledge about the physiological basis of optimism and happiness (explored in Chapter 2) can inform practical approaches for improving our resilience and coping skills in the face of hardship, our emotional and social intelligence, and our sense of well-being (Chapter 3).[9] These changes, in turn, enhance cognitive performance and help us to be more creative and more successful at work, to have more fulfilling relationships, and to enjoy better health.

2. **Become functionally smarter for higher levels of achievement.** Our collective IQ, through the so-called *Flynn effect*, has increased over the last century, and we can continue to improve our individual intellectual performance by cultivating cognitive and metacognitive strategies. This purposeful approach to enhancing our thinking abilities, which we call *practical metacognition*, can help us learn new things more efficiently, make better decisions, solve problems more effectively, and create new ideas. The increase in cognitive skills, sense of efficacy, and success in school, in work, and in life pays an added dividend in the form of increased levels of optimism and happiness. Chapters 4 through 6 explore findings from mind, brain, and education research on "working smarter" by wielding cognitive and metacognitive strategies and improving your social intelligence with the aim of enhancing achievement and success.

3. **Improve physical well-being, mood, and cognitive function through exercise and healthy nutrition.** In Chapters 7 and 8, we explore how healthy eating and regular exercise bolster physical and cognitive performance and improve mood and outlook. Making a habit of aerobic exercise, strength training, and good nutrition can produce lifelong health gains. In addition, exercise changes the brain in positive ways and is effective in improving mood. Regular physical activity is associated with improved quality of sleep, reduced fatigue, increased stamina, and lower anxiety. For some people, exercise may be as effective as medications in the longer term to treat mood disorders. A stronger body is also associated with enhanced cognitive performance in areas such as attention, memory, and problem solving.

All of these factors can be enhanced individually, and greater gains can be experienced through the synergy of improving them together so that we can become positively smarter, fitter, stronger, and better able to achieve important goals while experiencing a greater sense of well-being.

The capacity to realize higher levels of happiness, achievement, and physical health begins with your amazing brain, powered by some 86 billion neurons. Just one cubic centimeter of your brain has as many connections as there are stars in the Milky Way.[10] Scientists have learned more about the brain in the last two decades than in the previous 200 years. These discoveries can have a positive and far-reaching impact on our lives, our work, our education, and our communities if and when these new understandings are used to inform policy and practice.

At the center of emerging scientific knowledge is one fundamental concept: Your brain and body are constantly changing in response to your thoughts, actions, and environment, and you have the power to steer those changes in positive directions. You can take charge of your thinking, attitudes, and behaviors in ways that affect:

- Neurogenesis, the creation of new brain cells;
- Synaptogenesis, the forging of new connections and strengthening or weakening of networks of connections as a result of learning new knowledge or skills;
- Myelination, the formation of a substance that insulates and increases the speed of transmission of new learning and improves skills; and
- Angiogenesis, the expansion of your body's network of capillaries to improve the functioning of the brain and body.

We refer to the dynamic interactions that influence these factors as *neurocognitive synergy* to convey that through your conscious (or *cognitive*) recognition of your ability to take charge of your brain (*neuro*), you can wield a game-changing combination (*synergy*) to become more optimistic, functionally smarter and more productive, and healthier.

The research behind this concept informs, in part, the emerging field of educational neuroscience, which melds psychological and educational research and cognitive neuroscience to explore ways for enhancing teaching and learning. These findings also offer great promise to improve our personal and professional lives. Throughout this book, we will explore the research advances supporting the understanding that it is within your grasp to make steady gains if you are willing to commit to the sometimes hard work of deliberate practice, the learning of new knowledge, and the process of maintaining a happier outlook, developing your cognitive skills, and improving your physical well-being. These "upgrades" in attitude, thinking, and health habits in turn serve to sustain the behaviors that can have a positive influence in many areas of your life.

Learning about the brain's awesome power that can help each of us develop the knowledge and skills we need to achieve our goals is crucial. But to use that power to optimize our potential, we need to bring to the surface some deeply held misconceptions that may be holding us back.

Our Personal Introductions to the Science That Supports Ways for Becoming Positively Smarter

Our work together has focused on improving lives by applying the implications of research from fields including cognitive education; psychology; social cognitive and affective neuroscience; education; and well-being. We are codevelopers of curriculum for the master's and educational specialist degrees with majors in brain-based teaching and a doctoral minor in brain-based leadership with Nova Southeastern University. These programs are among the first in this emerging field, also known as educational neuroscience and mind, brain, and education.[11] The principles at the core of this text have informed our work on the graduate degree programs and the presentations we have delivered through the Center for Innovative Education and Prevention.

Earlier in his career, Marcus applied research from these diverse fields in his work with organizations from business, law enforcement, military, government, and education sectors. He led a three-year, statewide initiative for the Florida Department of Education, implementations in two large school districts through Florida Atlantic University supported by an Annenberg Challenge Grant, a statewide initiative in Texas, and an implementation on improving well-being with the Winter Park Health Foundation. Marcus has continued to discuss the ideas and research at the heart of becoming positively smarter as an author and international speaker on increasing creative and critical thinking skills, developing expertise, and enhancing achievement and well-being.

Donna began her career as a classroom teacher and then an educational and school psychologist who completed post-doctoral studies in structural cognitive modifiability. She led an initiative in her school district to teach students how to use cognitive strategies—to "learn how to learn"—which resulted in significant academic gains. Co-teaching these concepts with other educators led Donna to discover her passion for working as a teacher educator. In the intervening years, she has led community and district initiatives and given presentations to state and national

8

policymakers that put some key concepts from this book into practice.

Our aim is to highlight ways research and theory from cognitive education, psychology, and educational neuroscience suggest that we can harness the brain's incredible capacity to change in ways that may enhance resilience, optimism, motivation, happiness, productivity, performance, and well-being. If you set your sights on any of these areas, you can achieve benefits through the sustained application of practical strategies. The grand vision of becoming positively smarter is informed by research about the interconnections of emotional and physical health and cognitive performance: It is possible to make gains in all of these areas and create a positive upward spiral that can produce positive changes in the brain and in turn lead to a greater sense of well-being.

Our perspective is from the field of education, and our focus is on sharing relevant research and practical ideas for putting implications of research into practice. We have assembled here emerging, exciting findings from a broad range of scientific inquiry to discover how each of us can achieve more of our unique potential to become happier and healthier and achieve more of our personal and professional goals. The practical applications we have shared with educators, parents, businesspeople, firefighters, police officers, military members, and others in helping professions begin with a stunning fact: Our capacity to become happier, functionally smarter, and healthier begins with our marvelous, malleable brains.

Notes

1 Eric R. Kandel. 2007. "The New Science of Mind." *Best of the Brain from Scientific American*. New York: Dana Press. Retrieved from https://faculty.washington.edu/chudler/quotes.html

2 Harvard-Smithsonian Center for Astrophysics. 1987. *A Private Universe* [DVD]. Cambridge, MA: Author.

3 Robert L. Sternberg, Linda Jarvin, and Elena L. Grigorenko. 2009. *Teaching for Wisdom, Intelligence, Creativity, and Success*. Thousand Oaks, CA: Corwin Press, p. 4.

4   Heidi Grant Halvorson. 2012. *Succeed: How We Can Reach Our Goals.* New York: Plume, p. 215.

5   Carol Dweck. 2006. *Mindset, the New Psychology of Success: How We Can Learn to Fulfill Our Potential.* New York: Ballantine.

6   M. J. A. Howe, J. W. Davidson, and J. A. Sloboda. *Innate Gifts and Talents: Reality or Myth?* p. 2. Retrieved from http://users.ecs.soton. ac.uk/harnad/Papers/Py104/howe.innate.html

7   K. Anders Ericsson and Neil Charness. "Expert Performance: Its Structure and Acquisition." *American Psychologist, 49*(8), August 1994, 725–747.

8   Tali Sharot, Alison M. Riccardi, Candace M. Raio, and Elizabeth A. Phelps. "Neural Mechanisms Mediating Optimism Bias." *Nature, 450,* November 1, 2007, 102–105.

9   Richard J. Davidson, with Sharon Begley. 2012. *The Emotional Life of Your Brain.* New York: Hudson Street Press, pp. 10–11.

10   David Eagleman. 2012. *Incognito: The Secret Lives of the Brain.* New York: Pantheon, p. 2.

11   Sarah D. Sparks. "Experts Call for Teaching Educators Brain Science." *Education Week, 31*(33), June 4, 2012. Retrieved from http://www. edweek.org/ew/articles/2012/06/06/33teachers.h31.html

1

Building a Smarter Brain

"Brain plasticity is the stuff of life. As long as you're alive, it's with you as a precious exploitable asset. Don't neglect to take full advantage of it."
—Michael Merzenich[1]

No matter what your age or current abilities, you have the potential to improve the knowledge and skills you need to develop to achieve your goals—in the form of your brain's amazing ability to change in response to learning. Recent research is overturning longstanding assumptions about the capacity of the human brain to change and improve. We now know that people, with the exception of some of those who have suffered traumatic brain injury, dementia, or other brain disorder, have the capability to change and grow their brains, especially those areas of the brain associated with attention, memory, and problem solving. These are the very areas we associate with becoming smarter. The term *neural plasticity* or *neuroplasticity* refers to how our thoughts, actions, and sensory input (what we see, hear, say, and touch) change the structure and function of the brain and how reinforcing that learning through repetition and practice strengthens those neural connections. When we focus our attention on information and engage in

Positively Smarter: Science and Strategies for Increasing Happiness, Achievement, and Well-Being, First Edition. Marcus Conyers and Donna Wilson.

learning activities, the neural networks associated with those activities grow denser and larger, leading to what Fotuhi describes as "enhanced brain performance."[2] In fact, these physical changes in the brain can be so significant that they can be seen by the human eye on MRI scans—and these changes can happen in weeks and months, rather than years.

Neuroplasticity in Action

In a regimen unlike any other in the world, London cabbies in training spend years memorizing their city's 25,000 streets and thousands of landmarks within a 6-mile radius of Charing Cross train station. Some of them take the Knowledge of London Examination, known simply as "the Knowledge," a dozen times, and only about half ultimately earn an operating license from the Public Carriage Office.[3] Neurologists Katherine Woollett and Eleanor Maguire conducted MRI brain scans of 79 taxi trainees and a control group before the training began and again three or four years later after they had completed their exams. Of the three groups during the second round of testing—trainees who had earned their licenses, trainees who had not passed the exam, and control participants—the scans detected an increase in gray matter volume in the posterior hippocampi, the area of the brain associated with spatial memory, of the first group, but not the other two. The researchers concluded that "specific, enduring, structural brain changes in adult humans can be induced by biologically relevant behaviors engaging higher cognitive functions."[4]

The cabbie research is among a number of studies conducted in recent years that show how the brain changes in response to learning. German scientists conducted brain imaging scans of medical students three months before their medical exams and immediately following the tests and compared them to scans of a control group of students. The brains of the medical students showed increased volume in areas of their parietal cortices and the posterior hippocampi, regions of the brain associated with memory retrieval and learning.[5] Another study compared the brains of professional musicians who practiced with their instruments at least an hour per day to the brains of amateur musicians and non-musicians. The scans showed significant increases in gray matter volume in brain regions associated with motor, auditory, and visual-spatial functioning of the professional musicians in comparison with the other groups; amateur musicians also showed more development in these regions than non-musicians. The researchers concluded that those differences reflect the impact of "long-term skill acquisition and the repetitive rehearsal of those skills."[6] These studies demonstrate neuroplasticity in action as the brain changes in response to learning new knowledge and developing skills. They also disprove long-held assumptions that adult brains cannot build new neurons.

Other research challenges the notion that IQ is unchangeable—that we are born with a certain level of intelligence and cannot "move the dial" on our intellectual capacity. As it turns out, that notion may be wrong on both counts: Research now suggests that we can increase our intelligence throughout life and that heredity may account for only a relatively small portion of our cognitive potential. By conducting DNA analysis and comparing IQ test results from people tested at age 11 and again when they were 65 to 79, Scottish researchers concluded that only about 24 percent of intellectual development is determined by genes; the rest owes to one's experiences and environment throughout life.[7] In another study, 33 adolescents ages 12 to 16 took IQ tests and underwent brain scans in 2004 and then repeated the tests three or four years later, now at ages 15 to 20. There were no cognitive interventions or tests between the two periods; in fact, the teenagers were not even told they would be invited back for further testing. The researchers' aim was to measure whether intellect, as measured by the Wechsler Intelligence Scale for children and adults, would change and to see if IQ changes would be reflected in brain structure. They discovered significant shifts up and down in IQ—ranging from a drop of 20 points for one participant to a gain of 23 points for another in verbal IQ, a range of −18 to +17 in performance IQ (nonverbal skills, including spatial reasoning and problem solving unrelated to language), and a range of −18 to +21 in full-scale IQ—along with corresponding changes in gray matter density and volume in the brain scans.[8]

Scientists have varying opinions about what IQ tests tell us about people's intellectual capacity. These differences of opinion are evident in debates over what causes the "Flynn effect," the steady rise in IQ levels around the world since the 1930s, which was first identified by New Zealand political science professor James Flynn. Are today's students really smarter than their grandparents, or are they just better test takers? Some social scientists attribute these IQ gains to the wider availability of public education, the increase in years spent in formal education, and even on improved nutrition. Others suggest that IQ tests evolve with each generation to emphasize the skills most prized during that era. Still others argue that this trend calls into question the reliability of IQ tests in measuring "pure" intelligence.

As we will explore in more detail later in this chapter, intelligence is multifaceted—and people have the capacity to improve many aspects of their intellectual functioning, including creativity, analytical problem solving, recall, and mental agility. In sum, then, the conclusion we can draw from this research on the mind and brain, notes Edward Hallowell in his book *Shine: Using Brain Science to Get the Best from Your People*, is that "we can all get smarter and wiser and happier the longer we live. The conventional, dreary wisdom that people can't change is scientifically incorrect."[9]

Your Brain at Work: A Continual Construction Zone

As the control center in charge of all aspects of operating a living creature—from controlling basic functions such as heart rate and breathing to accepting and interpreting input from the senses to facilitating thought and experiencing emotions—the brain is understandably complex. As we explore the role of the brain in our efforts to improve our positive outlook, knowledge, skills, and well-being, we will present research findings on the workings of the cerebral cortex and the limbic system. The *cerebral cortex* is the

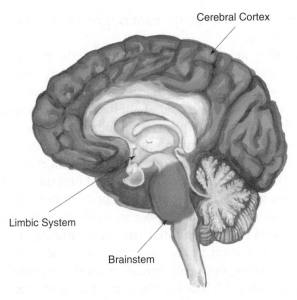

Figure 1.1 A Three-Part Brain Model. © 2015 BrainSMART, Inc.

outer surface of the human brain that grows so extensively that it folds in on itself in labyrinth fashion, giving it a cauliflower appearance. The largest part of the brain is the neocortex, so named because it is the newest part of the human brain (the terms *cerebral cortex*, *cortex*, and *neocortex* are often used interchangeably). In his book *Boost Your Brain*, Majid Fotuhi describes the cortex as "ground zero for … perceptual awareness, thought, language, and ability to make decisions."[10] The *limbic system* is located directly under the cortex and shares several structures with the cortex. A third major region is the brainstem, which connects the brain to the spinal cord (see Figure 1.1).

The brain reflects the symmetry of the human body: We have two eyes, two ears, two arms, two legs, and two hemispheres of the cerebral cortex. The right and left hemispheres are connected by a band of nerve fibers called the corpus callosum. The right hemisphere controls most motor functions on the left side of the body, while the left hemisphere controls the right side. That's why a stroke or other type of brain damage in the left hemisphere may hamper motor function on the right side of the face, the right arm, and the right leg.

Though they are near mirror structures, the two hemispheres have some specialized functions. Areas of the left hemisphere are associated with language, math, and logic processing, while the right hemisphere supports spatial abilities, facial recognition, and myriad other functions. But even though some thinking abilities seem to be more dominant in one hemisphere or the other, both sides are involved in most complex cognitive processes. For example, one of the left hemisphere's specialized functions is helping to decipher sounds that form words and applying the rules of syntax to find meaning in the order of words, while the right hemisphere is more attuned to the emotional aspects of language conveyed by rhythm and intonation.[11] The two hemispheres also play differing roles in modulating optimistic and pessimistic responses to external stimuli, with the left hemisphere exhibiting greater activation in positive interactions and the right hemisphere more active in situations involving stress, fear, and negative emotions.[12] These findings underscore that emotions are not just fleeting states but have a biological component.

The hemispheric division provides additional evidence of the brain's plasticity in action. In several much-studied cases, neurologists disconnected the brain hemispheres to eliminate debilitating seizures in patients with severe epilepsy. With extensive support and therapy, these patients have, to varying degrees, been able to "retrain" their brains to take over some of the functions previously handled by one or the other hemisphere. The fact that the brain can so extensively rewire itself demonstrates that "the brain is far more malleable than we once thought."[13]

Each hemisphere of the cortex is further divided into four lobes (see Figure 1.2); these paired lobes have specialized functions:

- The *frontal lobes*, located behind and just above the eyes in front of the central sulcus (a deep groove in both hemispheres that separates the frontal and parietal lobes), are the centers of planning, decision making, problem solving, and control of body

16

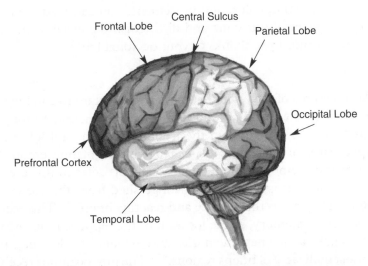

Figure 1.2 The Four Brain Lobes. © 2015 BrainSMART, Inc.

movements. The *prefrontal cortex*, located directly behind the forehead, is interconnected to every distinct functional unit of the brain and thus coordinates and integrates most brain functions. Often referred to as the brain's "CEO" or "conductor," this region is essential to both foresight, which is necessary for rational, logical thought, and the insight required for empathy and social skills.[14] The prefrontal lobes are also the area of the brain that undergo the most extensive postnatal development.[15]

- The *temporal lobes*, on each side of the skull, are the centers for processing what we hear, smell, and taste. These lobes help us understand verbal communications and other auditory input and play a role in higher-level visual processing as well.[16]
- The *parietal lobes*, located between the frontal and occipital lobes and just above the temporal lobes, aid in navigation, the processing of tactile sensations (or input from our skin), and the orientation of our body and limbs.
- The *occipital lobes*, along the back section of the cortex, are the brain's visual processing center, responsible for the recognition

of shape, depth, color, and movement. You can read the print on the pages of this book and distinguish the facial features of people around you thanks to your occipital lobes.

Another area of the brain that plays an important role in how we interact with the world around us is the *limbic system,* a group of interconnected structures in the frontal and temporal lobes and deeper parts of the brain associated with regulating emotional activity and memory.[17] Some neuroscientists refer to this area as the *limbic lobe*; it is sometimes distinguished from the cortex, or "thinking brain," as the "feeling and reacting brain."[18] This region is also key to memory, as the location of the hippocampus, which is "the gateway for new memories and essential for learning [as] the most malleable of brains regions."[19] The hippocampus receives input from throughout the neocortex and the limbic system.

The limbic system is also home to the amygdala, a paired structure in each brain hemisphere with reciprocal connections to many parts of the brain. The amygdala causes that startle response we have to external stimuli we might perceive as threatening, which gives it the nickname "fear button." When it detects the potential for danger, the amygdala immediately signals another structure in the limbic system, the hypothalamus, to take protective action (fight or flight). The frontal lobes also receive signals from the amygdala and process whether the stimuli represents a real threat. When you see a slender object in the grass next to your walking path, for example, the amygdala may sound the alarm of "Snake!" until the frontal lobes process the input and respond, "Nope, just a stick."

New imaging technologies have been useful in pinpointing the functions of these various structures—and in furthering our understanding of the brain's plasticity. How does your brain form new neurons and synapses, and is there anything you can do to optimize those processes? Several functions are at work to power the neurocognitive synergy that supports learning, recall, and the development of knowledge and skills. Fotuhi refers to the "Core 4" of growing your brain: increasing the number of brain cells, adding synapses, bolstering neuronal connections through myelination, and enhancing blood flow in the body and brain.[20]

Neurogenesis The most basic operating units of the brain are neurons, nerve cells that transmit signals in the form of electrical impulses. For much of the previous century, many scientists believed *neurogenesis,* or the creation of new neurons, to be a function of young brains; this view held adulthood to be a period of steady, inevitable decline in the number of brain cells and, thus, of brain function. A major epiphany in the 1980s was accompanied by bird song, as researchers reported that the brains of adult songbirds formed new neurons as they learned new songs.[21] It seems that you can teach an old bird new songs just as you can teach an old dog new tricks—and both of their brains form new neurons as a result of that learning!

In the years since those findings of neurogenesis in adult brains, there has been an explosion of research about what regulates the formation and development of human brain cells, from the actions of stress hormones called glucocorticoids that appear to impair neuronal production to brain chemicals like BDNF (discussed later in this chapter) that support brain growth. For example, through their research focusing on the hippocampus, Fotuhi and his colleagues have found that it is possible to "not only reverse the brain atrophy associated with aging but also expand the brain's size—even before shrinkage begins."[22] The key is to make the most of the new neurons that form regularly by taking "brain-healthy" actions that enhance neuronal survival.

Synaptogenesis Neurons form neural networks through "synaptic connections" between the cells; the more activity is transmitted through those networks, the stronger the connections. However, when these connections are not reinforced with regular stimuli, they are weakened and ultimately eliminated. The formation of neural connections is known as *synaptogenesis,* while decreases in those networks are referred to as *pruning.* Pruning may sound like a bad thing, but it's a natural and useful process that ensures that the brain operates efficiently. Both of these processes are behind the structural changes that encode learning and memories in the brain, and they are essential in continually developing the skills and knowledge you need to accomplish the goals you set for yourself.

A primary force at work in developing new knowledge and skills is *experience-dependent synaptogenesis*, the formation of synaptic connections in response to our experiences and environment. These connections don't just form naturally; they are not an automatic product of getting another year older and more mature. Instead, they are a direct result of what we hear, see, taste, smell, do, and think. And the more we think about or do something, the stronger these connections get. Experience-dependent synaptogenesis is behind the learning that results when we expand our vocabulary, take up a new hobby like knitting or woodworking, practice a new piece of music on our instrument of choice, or become familiar with the rhythm of a dance step. It happens because we decide to learn something new, commit the time and effort to do so, and have the proper conditions and resources, such as a good coach or pertinent information, for learning.

Myelination The brain consists of both gray matter, which is primarily neurons, and "white matter," or myelin produced by glial cells and interspersed among neurons to insulate and support neural connections. Myelin, which is composed of fats, protein, and water, is an electrical conductor that increases the speed and strength of the impulses transmitted among neurons. Adequate myelination supports healthy brain and body functioning; conversely, a breakdown in the myelination process, or demyelination in the brain and spinal cord, is a factor in multiple sclerosis (MS) and other diseases that cause nervous system degeneration.

Angiogenesis Blood vessels supply oxygen and nutrients to your body and brain, and the development of new blood vessels, called *angiogenesis*, helps maintain the blood supply to the brain. A healthy diet, rich in fruits and vegetables, and regular exercise enhance the development of new blood vessels for peak functioning of your body–brain system.

Beyond Conventional Wisdom: Harnessing Your Neurocognitive Synergy

These four processes combine to contribute to the brain's peak functioning. And in terms of the aim to become positively smarter, a key point is that we can take actions to enhance neurogenesis, synaptogenesis, myelination, and angiogenesis. The work of researchers around the world supports two essential aspects of the power of human potential: (1) our conscious choice to commit to the work of learning new information and skills changes the brain with the end result that (2) we can increase our marvelous, malleable intelligence and positive and productive outlook over time. As science writer Sharon Begley notes, these findings expand our understanding of the capacity of all people "to know more, to understand more deeply, to make greater creative leaps, to retain what we read, to see connections invisible to others—not merely to make the most of what we have between our ears now, but to be, in a word, smarter."[23]

Let's consider the implications of the exciting discoveries in recent decades about the brain processes that come together in neurocognitive synergy to support our capacity to become functionally smarter, achieve the goals we set for ourselves, and improve our well-being.

Intelligence Takes Many Forms

Since the dawn of the previous century, when Charles Spearman put forth the *g*-factor theory of intelligence as a single ability that applies to many different tasks, researchers from a variety of fields have continued to explore the nature of intelligence. Multifaceted conceptions put forth in the decades since hold that intelligence encompasses a variety of abilities, such as verbal comprehension and fluency, inductive reasoning, spatial visualization, and memory.[24] In the 1960s, psychologist Raymond Cattell and colleague John Horn described two forms of intelligence, crystallized and fluid:[25]

- *Crystallized intelligence* refers to the knowledge and skills we have learned and the ability to apply our knowledge and skills. Books we read and retain and every seminar or workshop we participate in adds to our crystallized intelligence. In our work, we read at least 150 books and articles each year that inform our approach to teacher education, and each adds to our "network of knowing" that is crystallized intelligence.
- *Fluid intelligence* is about applying what we know in novel situations. It is where the rubber meets the road in wielding cognitive flexibility and abstract thinking and using problem-solving skills in new circumstances. Fluid thinking is necessary in many work environments, in continuing education, and in life in a global, technologically advanced society.

Crystallized intelligence is generally acknowledged to increase with age. Emerging research suggests that fluid intelligence might also be enhanced in the adult brain.[26] In his book *Future Bright*, the late University of California Professor Michael Martinez wrote of the importance of an active lifestyle as we age. He suggested considering novel learning goals such as tackling a new area of study, pursuing a new career path, exploring the world through travel, or learning a new language as just a few of many possible strategies for maintaining and even improving cognitive abilities.[27]

In *Teaching for Wisdom, Intelligence, Creativity, and Success*, Robert Sternberg, Linda Jarvin, and Elena Grigorenko note that psychologists and educators who view intelligence as multifaceted also tend to believe that it is malleable, that we can become smarter through learning. They put themselves squarely in this camp, professing the belief

> that everyone has some initial abilities, and that these can be developed into competencies, and that these competencies can in turn

be honed into expertise. ... We believe that the key to success in the classroom—and in life more broadly—lies in a combination of intelligence, creativity, and wisdom.[28]

Connecting brain research to these theories of intelligence, a group of Canadian scientists captured MRI images of the brains of 16 participants taking a battery of a dozen tasks designed to test planning, reasoning, verbal, attentional, and working memory skills. Their finding that those tests engaged distinct brain networks led them to the conclusion that "intelligence is most informatively quantified in terms of not one but multiple distinct abilities."[29]

People of All Ages Have the Capacity to Improve Their Knowledge and Abilities

An extension of the limiting belief that intelligence is fixed is that current performance predicts future achievement. This belief is evident in the perception that children who begin school without having had the opportunity to develop preliteracy skills are destined for academic failure. It is true that early learning experiences matter: There is as much as a six-year difference in reading skills among kindergartners—from children who are already reading to those who don't yet know the basic mechanics of books (e.g., that English text is read from left to right in rows on a page from top to bottom)—and a four-year difference in understanding math concepts.[30] But that does not mean students at the low end of the achievement scale are doomed to perform below standards throughout their school careers. Almost all can catch up—and even thrive academically—with an education system that ensures effective teaching, formative assessments to identify extra help and reteaching they may need, parental and community support, and their own commitment to learning.

The same dynamic is true for adults. You may have shied away from certain intellectual pursuits and physical activities because "I've never been good at that sort of thing." Applying what you know now about neuroplasticity and learning new skills, you can see that you can get better!

What We Do Has a Greater Influence on How We Age Than Genetics

Our biology is not our destiny. In fact, according to medical research, our health as we age is only about 25 percent heritable.[31] That means three-fourths of the factors that affect health are environmental and largely within our control. Quality of diet, quantity of exercise, sleep regimen, regularity of preventative health care, and avoidance or existence of risk factors such as exposure to tobacco smoke and overconsumption of alcohol all influence our quality of health and life as we age. As one medical writer suggests, "life span, including maximum life span and healthy life span, can be extended."[32] Our biological clocks may be ticking, but we have a large degree of control over when health alarms begin to sound. We'll review the research and recommendations on nutrition and exercise for a long and healthy life in later chapters of this book.

Maintaining positive health habits also can help to stave off negative changes in aging brains. Neural connections are formed in the brain whenever we learn new information and skills and reinforce our newfound knowledge through practice and repetition. Regular exercise and healthy eating support angiogenesis to ensure adequate oxygenated blood flow to the brain. Exercise has also been shown to boost levels of BDNF (brain-derived neurotrophic factor), which facilitates neurogenesis and synaptogenesis in areas such as the hippocampus, which is associated with learning and memory, and the frontal lobes, which are the center for abstract thinking and executive decision making, such as planning, organization, and analysis.

How We Think Can Influence Our Health

If we believe that our diet and exercise regimen will yield positive results and if we believe we have the capability to achieve our health goals, we are more likely to do so. Harvard researchers conducted an experiment to demonstrate that "mind-set matters." Housekeepers at seven hotels were divided into two groups. Participants in the first group were told that their work is good exercise and qualifies under the Surgeon General's recommendations for a healthy lifestyle; participants in the control group did not hear this message. Four weeks later, the participants in the first group who believed that their work provided a healthy daily workout lost weight and lowered their blood pressure, body fat, waist-to-hip ratio, and body mass index.[33] This research shows that a positive outlook and being mindful of our health are useful components of a healthy lifestyle. As we will see in Chapter 4, determination and motivation also contribute to the role of thinking our way to better health.

We Can Build Muscle and Become Stronger Well into Our Eighties

Over the past decade, gerontologists and other medical doctors treating older adults have identified frailty as a diagnosable condition, characterized by fatigue, muscle loss, unintentional weight loss, and low levels of physical activity. But they stress that frailty is not an inevitable result of aging.[34] While many people lose muscle mass as they age, strength training offers the same benefits to middle-aged and older adults as it does to younger adults. In Chapter 7, we review the results of several studies of people in their 60s to 90s lifting weights and undergoing resistance training.

It's Hard to Identify the Children Who Are "Destined for Greatness"

The idea that it is easy to accurately predict which children will be future exceptional achievers in academics, athletics, art, and music represents a mindset that may actually do more harm than good for both "prodigies" and their "average" peers. Early high achievers may internalize the message that their accomplishments are the product of natural talent and dismiss the need for continual practice and learning to continue to build their knowledge and skills. Hearing the same message, their peers may give up trying to excel, accepting that they do not have the "gifts" required for success. The best-selling author Malcolm Gladwell was identified as a running prodigy as a teenager, but after competitive setbacks and a loss of interest, he stepped away from training. When he returned to running a few years later, he realized he was not an elite runner but "simply okay." In a 2006 speech at the Association for Psychological Science, Gladwell made the case that what sets gifted children apart is their dedication to learning. "Really what we mean ... when we say that someone is 'naturally gifted' is that they practice a lot, that they want to practice a lot, that they like to practice a lot."[35] The importance of deliberate practice in progressing toward the goals we set for ourselves is a major theme of Chapter 4.

Perceptions about Malleable vs. Fixed Intelligence Matter—a Lot

How we think about our ability to improve and succeed in achieving the goals we set for ourselves is at the heart of our chances of realizing our potential to become positively smarter. The persistent misconception that intellectual and physical abilities are inherent and cannot be improved holds people back, suggests Heidi Grant Halvorson in her book *Succeed*: "Decades of research suggest that the belief in fixed ability is completely wrong—abilities of all kinds are profoundly malleable. Embracing the fact that you can change will allow you to make better choices and reach your fullest potential."[36]

We have seen the power of this message—that you can become functionally smarter by putting in the effort to learn—resonate throughout our years working in education. As a school psychologist in Oklahoma earlier in her career, Donna assessed many students with learning challenges who made significant academic gains after they were taught that they could do better in school once they "learned how to learn" by using cognitive and metacognitive strategies (see Chapter 5).

A few years later, I had the opportunity to study at cognitive psychologist Reuven Feuerstein's institute, the International Center for the Enhancement of Learning Potential, in Jerusalem. Feuerstein's work dates back to the 1950s when he introduced a new approach to teaching young people who had survived the Holocaust and youth with Down syndrome and other disabilities. The academic progress these young people made is both inspiring and effective in beginning to dismantle the then-longstanding notion of fixed intelligence. Feuerstein looked past the subpar performance on IQ tests of young people who had lived through unspeakable horrors of World War II and lost their entire families, escaping with not even a photograph to remember them. Instead, he focused on their potential to learn and to regain a sense that some good could come into their lives. By offering intensive psychological and educational support, Feuerstein and his colleagues helped these young people recover from their losses, commit to their academic studies, and go on to become flourishing citizens. Introducing the concept of "structural cognitive modifiability," Feuerstein's work helped redefine intelligence not as a fixed attribute but as "the ability to learn."[37] He demonstrated that when teachers provide effective instruction and model an optimistic approach to learning, virtually all students can improve their intellectual performance. We mourned Professor Feuerstein's death in 2014, but his work has reverberated throughout recent decades in findings from other educational psychologists and researchers and will continue to inspire advances in educational practice.

As just one example, psychologist Carol Dweck has assembled a body of research behind the conception of a "growth mindset," or the belief that we can become smarter through education and effort.[38] In comparison, people with a fixed mindset believe intelligence is innate, and no amount of learning and hard work can enhance a person's IQ. As a result, children and adults with a fixed mindset tend to give up easily when faced with a learning challenge; they do not see a reason to work hard because they believe themselves to be limited in their intellectual capacity—thus creating a self-fulfilling prophecy. On the other hand, people with a growth mindset are motivated to work hard and persist in their efforts to learn new knowledge and skills because they know they can get better at whatever they set their minds to achieve.

Dweck and fellow researchers have tested their mindset theory in academic settings. In one study with seventh graders, students with a growth mindset consistently outperformed peers with a fixed mindset in math grades, and the gap in performance widened over the two years of the study.[39] This is one of several studies demonstrating that people who understand the concept of neuroplasticity and believe in the power of their personal potential can make significant gains through hard work and persistence.

These findings are borne out by the work of K. Anders Ericsson, who set out with colleagues in the early 1990s to determine what sets masters of their crafts and elite performers apart from peers in their chosen fields. Ericsson, Krampe, and Tesch-Romer identified several key elements of "deliberate practice" that lead to expert performance, including at least a decade of hard work; access to effective teachers and coaches, training materials, and facilities; adequate resources; and extraordinary commitment and motivation.[40] Along the way, these cognitive researchers also compiled extensive evidence to discount beliefs that expert performers, including celebrated musicians, elite artists, successful athletes, chess masters, and leading academics, relied primarily on innate talent to rise to the top of their professions. They trace the origins of attributing success to "natural abilities" back to the 19th century, but argue that "the differences between expert performers and normal adults reflect a life-long period of deliberate effort to improve performance in a specific domain."[41] We'll explore the concept of deliberate practice in more detail in Chapter 4, but for now, we underscore one essential conclusion that can be drawn from Ericsson's work: Gains in knowledge and skill are the result of hard work and persistence fueled by neuroplasticity, not innate talent.

Perceptions matter a great deal when it comes to the actualization of our potential to become positively smarter. Ericsson's research indicates how deeply rooted and longstanding these misperceptions are, and Dweck's work shows how such beliefs can derail potential on an individual level. We believe these misconceptions have a powerful negative influence on policy, practice, and ultimately the success and well-being of millions of people. When people underestimate their own capabilities and those of others—of students, of employees and colleagues, of children and parents—the result may be a collective waste of capacity to do great things. Our aim in writing this book is to set a new course in which all people recognize their potential to seize opportunities and achieve higher levels of performance through their own effort.

Plasticity as a Path to Becoming Positively Smarter

Using the positively smarter lens can help you internalize and optimize the process of enhancing neuroplasticity in your brain. The brain changes naturally in response to your experiences and environment. But you can take charge of "building a better brain" by steering your attention, thoughts, and actions in the right direction to achieve your personal and professional goals. In his book *Soft-Wired*, Michael Merzenich explores how neuroplasticity holds the key for developing "abilities that are the fundamental bases of a happy and fulfilling life for you."[42] The following list offers practical applications and actions you can take to make the most of your potential fueled by plasticity.

1. **What's good for the body is good for brain plasticity.** A nutritious diet, regular physical activity, and adequate sleep are both heart-happy and brain-happy habits that support angiogenesis to get needed oxygen to the brain, neurogenesis to create new neurons, synaptogenesis to forge neural connections, myelination to facilitate and strengthen those connections, and optimal brain activity.[43]
2. **A positive outlook combined with honing your selective attention (see Chapter 2) can enhance plasticity.** When you are engaged, alert, and motivated, the brain releases neurotransmitters that support plasticity.[44] According to Fotuhi, "maintaining a calm and focused mindset actually makes new blood vessels grow and the network of connections between

brain regions become stronger."[45] Consider your own experiences trying to learn something new or solve a problem when you were alert, engaged, focused on the task at hand, and feeling positive about the likely outcome. Now switch gears and think about a learning experience or problem you were faced with while feeling tired, distracted, disinterested, and not hopeful. Which in your experience was the most productive state of feeling and thinking?

3. **Plasticity enables an upward spiral of incremental progress and rewards for the hard work of learning new knowledge and skills.** The gains of successive learning form a platform for the next round of moving forward and over time increase your *brain reserve*, which "enhances brain performance now and results in a more resilient brain as you age."[46]

4. **Conscious effort to SAVE new information aids in long-term recall.** Merzenich uses the term *soft-wired* to underscore that the brain maintains the ability to learn new knowledge and skills throughout the life span but that without reinforcement, the neural connections forged by learning can be dismantled. In other words, learning is not hard-wired permanently into your neural circuits. As we will explore in more detail in Chapter 4, memorization is an essential trait in developing expertise. The more information you have stored in long-term memory, the more easily you can recall and apply it. Learning and applying memory strategies is an effective means of optimizing neuroplasticity. We rely on the metaphor of hitting the SAVE key[47] to describe the steps of transferring new learning from short-term memory into longer-term storage in the brain's memory banks:

> **See.** Employing the sense of sight aids retention. If you can see something—a demonstration or a diagram, for example—rather than just hearing or reading an explanation, you will be more likely to recall it. Here's an example: What do you remember more the first time you meet someone, the name or the face? Most people

remember the face because visual information is more easily received, retained, and recalled.

Associate. Connect new information to existing knowledge or use a *mnemonic*, a pattern of letters, ideas, or associations that assists in recall. SAVE is an example of a mnemonic, an acronym that sets out the steps of this memory strategy. Making associations is useful because it guides you to analyze new information and make sense of it, which enhances the neural connections formed by learning. Let's say the local library offers a lecture on new ideas for gardening designed to increase yield while decreasing watering requirements. An experienced gardener can associate the new recommendations with existing practices and thus be able to recall them better than someone who has never planted a garden.

Vividly savor emotional responses. Emotional responses enhance memory. If a lecturer shares a funny or moving story, you are more likely to remember the key points that story illustrates. Likewise, those "a-ha!" moments when the metaphorical light bulb goes off above your head when you puzzle out a solution to a tough problem or understand and apply a complex concept evoke strong positive emotions. Take a moment to savor those emotions and the learning that produced them—and your ability to recall that learning will be enhanced.

Experience. Learning that engages the senses—doing, seeing, hearing, smelling, and tasting—boosts recall. Watching a coach demonstrate a new skill is helpful, but doing it yourself puts your body and brain into a more productive learning mode. Adding a physical component to a memory task can also aid retention. A favorite strategy among audiences at our professional development sessions is called Ten Pegs.[48] We call out 10 random words—for instance, tomatoes, molasses, steak, orange, bananas, ice cream, mustard, string, band-aid, eggs—and ask teachers to recall them. Most remember three or four before their memory begins to falter. Then we ask them to stand and recite the words as they tap a different "peg" on their bodies: tomatoes—tap your head; molasses—touch your shoulders; steak—put your hand on your heart; orange—touch your belly; bananas—put your hands on your hips; and on down to "pegging" eggs with your toes. When we ask teachers to recall the list using pegs, many remember all 10 words! Think about how you can adapt this strategy for remembering important details and helping to "soft-wire" them into your memory.

5. **Repetition and practice make the most of the brain's plasticity.** Analyzing new information and applying it in different situations—in education, we call this "transferring the learning"—reinforces neural connections. For example, if you learn a new organizational strategy at work and apply it at home as well, you have successfully transferred that learning and added a new tool to your practical metacognition toolkit. Along the same lines, practicing a manual process, such as playing a musical instrument, or an athletic move becomes easier with repetition as your brain over time connects all the motor skills involved in that process so that it can direct your body to execute them adeptly. In other catchier words, "practice makes cortex," and once this knowledge or skill is integrated into your brain, you can retrieve it, apply it, and build on it.[49]

6. **If you don't use it, you may lose it.** Remember how the intensive practice and retention demands of memorizing the streets and landmarks of London bulked up the hippocampi of taxi drivers who had attained their operating licenses? You might think that years of studying and decades of applying "the Knowledge" while navigating the London labyrinth would result in permanent brain changes. But even in this extreme example, the researchers behind that study noted that this

pattern of hippocampal development was not as pronounced in the brains of retired cabbies, "hinting that any changes acquired through learning might be reversed or 'normalized' when the call on stored memory representations lessens."[50] Keeping essential knowledge and skills fresh in your mind requires ongoing practice and application.

7. **Mental rehearsal puts plasticity to work as well.** Thus far, we have focused on how external stimuli in the form of new information, sensory input, and experiences create and strengthen neural connections, but Davidson notes that "the brain can also change in response to messages generated internally—in other words, our thoughts and intentions. These changes can increase or decrease the amount of cortical real estate devoted to specific functions."[51] He cites both a physical and a mental example: As an athlete imagines and steps through in her mind the specific sequence of a complicated maneuver, "the regions of the motor cortex that control the required muscles expand."[52] Along the same lines, people can learn to control behaviors associated with obsessive-compulsive disorder by focusing their thoughts on quieting, or decreasing the activity, in the "worry circuit" of their brains.

8. **Plasticity encompasses both neuronal growth and pruning.** Merzenich explains how "positive and negative plasticity" work together:

> The brain's goal is simple. Its positive, connection-strengthening plasticity is increasing the power of connections on and between all the brain cells that fire together at each moment of time, burning in those changes only if their actions contribute to success. Its negative, connection-weakening plasticity is reducing the power of the connections coming into the machinery or from other neurons that did not fire at that important moment. ... Positive plastic brain changes work to create a brighter and sharper picture of what's happening. At the same time, negative plastic brain changes are erasing a little of that irrelevant and interfering haze or noise that frustrate the construction and recording of a clear picture.[53]

That dynamic of positive and negative plasticity may be the key to another finding in the London cabbie study. Though the taxi drivers who earned their operating licenses had a much better memory of street layouts and landmark locations than study participants in the control group, the cabbies had much poorer recall in tests on new visual information, such as complex figures, than the control group.[54] These findings tie back to the learning gains that result from developing your selective attention (see Chapter 3) so you can focus on acquiring the knowledge and skills necessary to achieve your goals.

9. **Plasticity applies to different forms of intelligence.** Building a better brain can help you improve your knowledge and abilities beyond the skills measured on a standard IQ test. A big-picture view of intelligence is that it encompasses "a person's ability to adapt to the environment and to learn from experience"[55] and "the ability to function well in response to obstacles in life [and] your ability to figure out ways to be successful."[56] In that light, you can set your mind to enhancing your creativity, communication and interpersonal skills, and other aspects of emotional intelligence. And you can look inward to develop a more positive outlook and enhance your resilience. Davidson shares several examples of how "the mind changes the brain" through cognitive-behavior therapy to treat obsessive-compulsive disorders and depression.[57]

These findings about neuroplasticity highlight the many ways your amazing brain can help you to become positively smarter—by forging and reinforcing neural connections to maintain a more optimistic approach to life (Chapters 2 and 3) and to hone the various forms of intelligence you need to thrive in your personal and professional lives (Chapters 4, 5, and 6). The fact that brain plasticity benefits from sustaining a healthy diet and regular exercise regimen (Chapters 7 and 8) rounds out the third component of our formula for becoming positively smarter and underscores the importance of tending to your mind, body, and brain.

A New Positive Paradigm

We can apply these findings about neuroplasticity by comparing two opposing paradigms framed by the ABCs—the assumptions, behaviors, and consequences—of how we think about our capacity to become positively smarter. What we think about our potential to achieve (our assumptions) influences how we act (our behaviors), and how we act leads to certain outcomes (consequences). The first paradigm is based on a view of human potential as relying on innate talent (IT), while the second is founded on a view of potential as present but untapped (UP).

The Innate Talent (IT) Paradigm

Assumptions

1. Our abilities and intellect are fixed and innate, largely the product of genetics.
2. Special talents are obvious early in life.
3. These talents and gifts develop with minimal effort.
4. Talent is limited to a fortunate few.

Behavior Child development, education, and workplace systems focus on identifying individuals with high levels of innate talent and providing a conducive environment to allow them to flourish. Fewer opportunities are offered to those assessed as having less innate talent.

Consequence Many individuals and groups are not provided with opportunities to learn and grow. They internalize the misconception that they lack the capacity to learn, to excel, and to succeed. This reduces their effort in striving to improve their skills and abilities. The Innate Talent Paradigm may have negative ramifications for those identified as talented as well. If they embrace the assumption that their innate gifts will develop naturally with minimal effort, they may fail to develop their true potential by putting in the hard work necessary to excel. Thus, the full consequences may be a massive achievement gap.

The Untapped Potential (UP) Paradigm

Assumptions

1. We have tremendous untapped potential, the product of the combination of genetic traits and environment.
2. Our intellect and abilities are malleable and improvable.
3. Our intellect and abilities can be enhanced through conscious effort over time.
4. The vast majority of people can get good or better at the abilities of their choosing with learning and practice.

Behavior Child development, education, and workplace systems focus on creating opportunities for all to develop their skills and abilities.

Consequence Many more people realize higher levels of achievement. More confident of their abilities to improve with effort, people put in the hard work necessary to do so—and receive encouragement from others (spouses, parents, teachers, coaches, etc.) in their endeavors. And they learn and employ useful strategies to help achieve their ambitious goals.

The UP Paradigm offers a formulation of our potential to become positively smarter that has the power to transform us as individuals and collectively as a culture, as a nation, and as a world of diverse peoples each with our own unique dreams and talents. What stands in its way? Or, as Robert Greenleaf asked in his classic book *Servant Leadership,* "Who is the enemy?" Greenleaf noted that many people lay the blame for the ills and unreasonableness that plague society at the door of "evil, stupidity, apathy, the 'system.'" He coined a resonant phrase to describe what limits so many people from achieving their full capacity—"fuzzy thinking on the part of good, intelligent, vital people, and their failure to lead."[58] We must dispel the "fuzzy thinking" that surrounds human potential if we are to realize our dreams.

We will return in the final chapter of this book to the transformational capacity of the UP Paradigm to frame our ability to become positively smarter. But first we will explore the practical aspects of a wide range of research on how we can enhance our happiness, achievement, and well-being.

Notes

1   Michael Merzenich. 2013. *Soft-Wired: How the New Science of Brain Plasticity Can Change Your Life* (2nd ed.). San Francisco: Parnassus, p. 214.

2   Majid Fotuhi. 2013. *Boost Your Brain: The New Art and Science Behind Enhanced Brain Performance.* New York: HarperOne, p. 4.

3   Mark Brown. "How Driving a Taxi Changes London Cabbies' Brains." *Wired,* December 9, 2011. Retrieved from http://www.wired.com/2011/12/london-taxi-driver-memory

4   Katherine Woollett and Eleanor A. Maguire. "Acquiring 'the Knowledge' of London's Layout Drives Structural Brain Changes." *Current Biology,* December 20, 2011, 2109–2114. Retrieved from http://www.ncbi.nlm.nih.gov/pmc/articles/PMC3268356/

5   B. Draganski, C. Gaser, G. Kempermann, H. G. Kuhn, J. Winkler, C. Buchel, and A. May. "Temporal and Spatial Dynamics of Brain Structure Changes During Extensive Learning." *The Journal of Neuroscience, 26*(23), 2006, 6314–6317.

6   Christian Glaser and Gottfried Schlaug. "Brain Structures Differ Between Musicians and Non-Musicians." *Journal of Neuroscience, 23*(27), October 8, 2003. Retrieved from http://www.jneurosci.org/content/23/27/9240.full

7   Medical Research Council. "Genetic Study Offers Clues to How Intelligence Changes Through Life." News, January 19, 2012. Retrieved from http://www.mrc.ac.uk/news-events/news/genetic-study-offers-clues-to-how-intelligence-changes-through-life/

8   S. Ramsden, F. M. Richardson, G. Josse, M. S. C. Thomas, and colleagues. "Verbal and Non-Verbal Intelligence Changes in the Teenage Brain." *Nature, 479,* November 3, 2011, 113–116.

9   Edward Hallowell. 2011. *Shine: Using Brain Science to Get the Best from Your People.* Boston: Harvard Review Press, p. 29.

10 Fotuhi, p. 15.

11 N. R. Carlson. 2007. *Physiology of Behavior* (9th ed.). New York: Pearson Education; D. C. Miller. 2007. *Essentials of School Neuropsychological*

Assessment. Hoboken, NJ: Wiley; Carl Zimmer. "Doublethink: The Slight Differences Between the Hemispheres May Soup up the Brain's Processing Power." *Discover Magazine Presents the Brain,* Spring 2011, 69–70.

12 David Hecht. "The Neural Basis of Optimism and Pessimism." *Experimental Neurobiology, 22*(3), September 2013, 173–199. doi: 10.5607/en.2013.22.3.173

13 Zimmer, p. 70.

14 Robert Sylwester. 2005. *How to Explain a Brain: An Educator's Handbook of Brain Terms and Cognitive Processes.* Thousand Oaks, CA: Corwin Press, pp. 69–70.

15 Rand Swenson. 2006. "The Cerebral Cortex," Chapter 11 in *Review of Clinical and Functional Neuroscience.* Hanover, NH: Darmouth Medical School. Retrieved from http://www.dartmouth.edu/~rswenson/NeuroSci/chapter_11.html

16 Sylwester, p. 82.

17 Sylwester, p. 93; Fotuhi, p. 15.

18 Swenson, "Limbic System," Chapter 9 in *Review of Clinical and Functional Neuroscience.* Retrieved from http://www.dartmouth.edu/~rswenson/NeuroSci/chapter_9.html

19 Fotuhi, p. 16.

20 Fotuhi, pp. 26–28.

21 David R. Riddle and Robin J. Lichtenwalner. 2007. "Neurogenesis in the Adult and Aging Brain." In D. R. Riddle (Ed.), *Brain Aging: Models, Methods and Mechanisms* (Chapter 6). Boca Raton, FL: CRC Press. Retrieved from http://www.ncbi.nlm.nih.gov/books/NBK3874/

22 Fotuhi, p. 26.

23 Sharon Begley. "Buff Your Brain: Want to Be Smarter in Work, Love, and Life?" *Newsweek,* January 9 and 16, 2012, p. 30.

24 Donna Wilson and Marcus Conyers. 2013. *Five Big Ideas for Effective Teaching: Connecting Mind, Brain, and Education Research to Classroom Practice.* New York: Teachers College Press, p. 70.

25 John L. Horn and Raymond Cattell. "Refinement and Test of the Theory of Fluid and Crystallized Intelligence." *Journal of Educational Psychology, 57*(5), 1966, 253–270.

26 Robert Sternberg. "Increasing Fluid Intelligence Is Possible After All." *Proceedings of the National Academy of Sciences USA, 105*(19), May 13, 2008, 6791–6792; S. M. Jaeggi, M. Buschkuehl, J. Jonides, and W. J. Perrig. "Improving Fluid Intelligence with Training on Working Memory." *Proceedings of the National Academy of Sciences USA, 105*(19), May 13, 2008, 6829–6833.

27 Michael E. Martinez. 2013. *Future Bright: A Transforming Vision of Human Intelligence.* New York: Oxford University Press, p. 39.

28 Robert Sternberg, Linda Jarvin, and Elena L. Grigorenko. 2009. *Teaching for Wisdom, Intelligence, Creativity, and Success.* Thousand Oaks, CA: Corwin Press, p. 5.

29 Adam Hampshire, Roger R. Highfield, Beth L. Parkin, and Adrian M. Owen. "Fractionating Human Intelligence." *Neuron, 76,* December 20, 2012, p. 1236.

30 Lynn Fielding, Nancy Kerr, and Paul Rosier. 2007. *Annual Growth for All Students: Catch-up Growth for Those Who Are Behind.* Kennewick, WA: New Foundation Press.

31 James W. Curtsinger. "Genes, Aging, and Prospects for Extended Life Span." *Minnesota Medicine,* October 2007. Retrieved from http://www.minnesotamedicine.com/Past-Issues/Past-Issues-2007/October-2007/Clinical-Curtsinger-October-2007

32 Ibid.

33 Alia J. Crum and Ellen J. Langer. "Mind-Set Matters: Exercise and the Placebo Effect." *Psychological Science, 18*(2), 2007, p. 165.

34 Marlene Cimons. "Frailty Is a Medical Condition, Not an Inevitable Result of Aging." *The Washington Post,* December 10, 2012.

35 Eric Wargo. "The Myth of Prodigy and Why It Matters." *Observer, 19*(8), August 8, 2006. Retrieved from http://www.psychologicalscience.org/index.php/video/the-myth-of-prodigy-and-why-it-matters.html

36 Heidi Grant Halvorson. 2012. *Succeed: How We Can Reach Our Goals.* New York: Plume, p. 243.

37 Reuven Feuerstein, Raphael S. Feuerstein, Louis Falik, and Yaacov Rand. 2002. *Dynamic Assessments of Cognitive Modifiability.* Jerusalem, Israel: ICELP Press, p. 4.

38 Carol Dweck. 2006. *Mindset, the New Psychology of Success: How We Can Learn to Fulfill Our Potential.* New York: Random House.

39 L. S. Blackwell, K. H. Trzesniewski, and C. S. Dweck. "Implicit Theories of Intelligence Predict Achievement Across an Adolescent Transition: A Longitudinal Study and an Intervention." *Child Development, 78,* 2007, 256–263.

40 K. A. Ericsson, R. T. Krampe, and C. Tesch-Romer. "The Role of Deliberate Practice in the Acquisition of Expert Performance." *Psychological Review, 100*(3), 1993, 363–406.

41 Ericsson, Krampe, and Tesch-Romer, p. 400.

42 Merzenich, p. 59.

43 Fotuhi, pp. 30–33.

44 Merzenich, p. 53.

45 Fotuhi, p. 33.

46 Fotuhi, p. 34.

47 Donna Wilson and Marcus Conyers. 2011. *BrainSMART 60 Strategies for Increasing Student Learning* (4th ed.). Orlando, FL: BrainSMART, pp. 197–199.

48   Wilson and Conyers, pp. 294–295.
49   Emma G. Duerden and Daniele Laverdure-Dupont. "Practice Makes Cortex." *Journal of Neuroscience, 28*(35), 2008, 8655.
50   Woollett and Maguire.
51   Richard J. Davidson, with Sharon Begley. 2012. *The Emotional Life of Your Brain*. New York: Hudson Street Press, p. 162.
52   Ibid.
53   Merzenich, p. 58.
54   Woollett and Maguire.
55   Robert J. Sternberg. "Academic Intelligence Is Not Enough. WICS: An Expanded Model for Effective Practice in School and Later in Life." Paper commissioned for the Conference on Liberal Education and Effective Practice, March 12–13, 2009, p. 2. Retrieved from http://www.clarku.edu/aboutclark/pdfs/sternberg_wics.pdf
56   Fotuhi, p. 35.
57   Davidson, p. 172.
58   Robert K. Greenleaf. 2002. *Servant Leadership: A Journey into the Nature of Legitimate Power and Greatness* (25th anniversary edition), ed. Larry C. Spears. New York: Paulist Press, p. 58.

2

Why Happiness Matters

"Happy individuals are more likely than their less happy peers to have fulfilling marriages and relationships, high incomes, superior work performance, community involvement, robust health, and a long life."
—William Compton and Edward Hoffman[1]

For the vast majority of people in cultures around the world, achieving greater happiness is their foremost goal.[2] *Everyone*, for the most part, wants to be happy.

Though most everyone *wants* to be happy, maintaining a positive outlook, appreciating life's blessings, and being resilient in the face of setbacks most of the time day in and day out can be a challenge for many of us. Surprisingly, the things we believe will make us happy—be it more income, a new job, a new relationship, or more material possessions such as a new car—have only a short-term impact on the way we feel. As a result, we may come to regard happiness as a fleeting emotion outside of our control.

Nearly everyone wants to be *happy*, but what, exactly, does that mean? This confluence of a near-universal desire for happiness and confusion over how to achieve it has led to serious scientific study into what once might have been considered a frivolous pursuit. In

Positively Smarter: Science and Strategies for Increasing Happiness, Achievement, and Well-Being, First Edition. Marcus Conyers and Donna Wilson.

recent years, the United Nations has even published a *World Happiness Report* bringing together global survey data and research on the impact of subjective well-being on mental and physical health.[3]

Research has turned up some counterintuitive findings about the nature of happiness—how it can change our lives, what tools we have and can develop to achieve it, and why it is so crucial to do so. Discoveries from the fields of psychology and neuroscience—even from economics and political science—are providing concrete answers about how to find what so many people say they want more of in their lives.

Reaping the Many Benefits of Happiness

As if happiness were not its own reward—and it is certainly is that—maintaining an upbeat, optimistic outlook also makes a substantial positive difference in many aspects of our lives. Psychologist Richard Davidson sets out the various connections between how we feel and how well we think:

> When positive emotion energizes us, we are better able to concentrate, to figure out the social networks at a new job or new school, to broaden our thinking so we can creatively integrate diverse information, and to sustain our interest in a task so we can persevere.[4]

When we feel good:

- **We are more creative thinkers and better problem solvers.** In her book *Positivity*, psychologist Barbara Fredrickson refers to this connection as the "broaden-and-build" theory, setting out evidence that positive emotions "broaden people's ideas about possible actions, opening our awareness to a wider range of thoughts and actions than is typical ... [and] making us more receptive and more creative."[5] Creativity is a useful skill in our everyday lives and is increasingly prized in the workplace. In fact, creativity and openness to new ideas are among the top attributes that companies seek in new employees.[6]

- **We have stronger relationships.** Positive relationships with family, friends, colleagues, neighbors, and others with whom we interact on a daily basis are both a cause and effect of happiness. In his book *Flourish*, Martin Seligman sums up the research that we humans are social creatures down to our evolutionary roots—that the need to solve social problems required to live, work, and thrive alongside others created an anatomical characteristic that sets us apart from other species: "the big brain is a relationship simulation machine, and it has been selected by evolution for exactly the function of designing and carrying out harmonious but effective human relationships."[7] Moving forward in time to the present day, Seligman observes that "very little that is positive is solitary. ... *Other people* are the best antidote to the downs of life and the single most reliable up."[8] Positive relationships and interactions are a primary source of pleasure—of laughter, relaxation, and comfort—for happy people. We will explore the implications of our "social brains" in more depth in Chapter 6.

- **We perform better on the job and in our personal pursuits.** A *Wall Street Journal* study reports that happy employees are twice as productive as coworkers who focus on the negative. "Happier workers help their colleagues 33% more than their least happy colleagues; raise issues that affect performance 46% more; achieve their goals 31% more and are 36% more motivated."[9] Along the same lines, workplace studies by British researchers found that happy employees are 12 percent more productive than coworkers with a negative affect.[10] In addition to two commonly cited traits that determine high performance on the job—ability and motivation—economist Peter Schulman adds a vital third, an optimistic belief that you will achieve your goals: "The ability to succeed and the desire to succeed are not always enough without the belief that one will succeed. Someone with the talent of a Mozart can come to nothing in the absence of that belief. This is particularly true when the task at hand is challenging and requires persistence to overcome obstacles and setbacks."[11] In studies testing the impact of an optimistic mindset, salespeople maintaining a positive outlook outsold their more pessimistic coworkers by 20 to 40 percent across a variety of industries. This connection between a positive outlook and work success is important from the very beginning of one's career: Happy people are more likely to get second job interviews![12]

- **We are physically healthier.** A wide range of medical studies have concluded that an optimistic outlook—in particular the feeling that life is worth living—has a protective effect against cardiovascular disease. Three possible mechanisms connect happiness to physical health: (1) optimists, believing that they can make a difference, take action to maintain a healthy lifestyle; (2) they can rely on family and friends for social support; and (3) there may be biological mechanisms that shield optimists from serious illness or aid in their recovery.[13] We will explore the connection between physical health and happiness—and optimizing both—in later chapters of this book.

- **We are more resilient.** We find truly inspiring evidence of the power of a positive approach to help people cope with devastating events. Viktor Frankl's classic book, *Man's Search for Meaning,* relates how he found the strength to survive in the Auschwitz concentration camp by imagining a happier future.[14] The PBS special *Happy* shares the story of a former beauty queen who relied on her positive outlook to emerge from years of surgery and medical treatment following a disfiguring accident to settle into a new marriage and career. We will profile several people in later chapters who, after suffering personal tragedies, went on to create foundations and programs to make a positive difference for others. Developing and maintaining an optimistic outlook can put you on a "trajectory that cuts through dark times and leads you back to higher ground, stronger than ever."[15]

- **We benefit from a positive feedback loop.** Happiness begets more of the same: Happy people are more creative, more positive in their interactions with others, and thus more productive and successful. This success makes them happier and builds their confidence and willingness and motivation to take on new challenges, which in turn results in greater achievement—and more reasons to be happy. As Teresa Aubele and Susan Reynolds write, "Feeling pleasure can be so stimulating for your brain that it is primed to respond to pleasure in a way that reinforces pleasure. Your brain offers rewards to steer you on a pathway to happiness, and you can offer your brain rewards that will encourage it to become even more finely tuned—and to grow well into your old age."[16]

A positive outlook can elevate every aspect of our lives, producing a powerful, upward spiral. Success leads to greater happiness, but psychologists conducting a meta-analysis of 225 papers involving more than 275,000 subjects conclude that the reverse may also be true: Happy people are more successful. "We discovered a vast number of correlational studies showing positive associations between happiness and successful outcomes within all of the major life domains (i.e., work, love, health). ... Happiness may, in many cases, lead to successful outcomes, rather than merely following from them."[17]

In sum, happiness frees our minds to focus on what matters most to us, to achieve our goals, to overcome obstacles, and to rebound from setbacks. So, how can we get happier?

I'll Be Happy When ...

Many people associate happiness with a particular milestone or event. They think, "I'll be happier when I get a new job or when I get my new business off the ground." Or, "Finding true love is my key to happiness." Or, "I won't be happy until we have a child." Or, "I'm confused and frustrated because I don't know what I want to do with my life. Contentment will come when I discover what I was born to do." Or, "I'm unhappy with my weight/my wrinkles/my marriage/our cramped living quarters/the bills overflowing in my mailbox. Once I lose weight/get a facelift/get a divorce/move to a bigger place/make more money, I will finally be happy."

45

There's nothing wrong with these goals and aspirations. Many are common pursuits; some are even admirable. The only problem is that attaining them will *not* make you substantially happier over the long term. You can find a better job, get married, have children, improve your health, and acquire greater wealth—all without moving your happiness dial significantly or permanently. At best, you may enjoy a brief boost in happiness after achieving these aims and then return to your previous level, what researchers call your happiness "set point."[18] What many people believe will have significant impact on their long-term happiness actually produces only a minimal, short-term effect.

Researchers studying happiness have focused on three general influences: (1) one's genetic or familial propensity toward a positive outlook; (2) personal circumstances (socioeconomic, family, career, and health status) and major life events, both positive and negative; and (3) one's ability to affect optimism vs. pessimism and positive vs. negative responses to people and events. In *The How of Happiness*, Sonja Lyubomirsky recounts her work with colleagues to quantify the impact of each of these areas. Based on studies with fraternal and identical twins, they conclude that the inherent set point for happiness, which had previously been viewed by many psychologists as the overwhelming influence, accounts for only about half of one's outlook. Another 10 percent is determined by differences in life circumstances—those milestones and events like getting married, getting a promotion, and buying a bigger house. Many people spend much of their lives in pursuit of things they believe will help them achieve happiness, when in reality those "big deals" don't move the dial on our happiness much after all.

The remaining 40 percent is within each person's control, offering the opportunity to adjust one's happiness set point up or down—"to increase or decrease our happiness levels through what we *do* in our daily lives and how we think."[19] One of the pillars of becoming positively smarter is to understand the factors in this "zone of opportunity" that can make you substantially happier over the long term and to invest your thinking and actions into making progress in these areas. You can become functionally smarter—and happier. Happiness and intelligence can both be cultivated through diligent effort, and growing one can have a positive impact on the other. That's excellent news because it means you don't have to wait until you double your salary or drop three dress sizes to feel happier. You can start right now. In Chapter 3, we offer 15 strategies to set you on that path.

What Is This Thing Called Happiness?

The fleeting feelings that many people think of as happiness are just one aspect of the state we are exploring in this book. Life is full of ups and downs. The ups run from simple pleasures to laugh-out-loud exhilarations, and the downs range from minor annoyances to major catastrophes. How we respond emotionally to those experiences arises from a complex interplay of influences dictated by:

- **Our brain chemistry.** The brain produces chemicals called *neurotransmitters* in response to both internal functions and external stimuli that affect how we feel. Chemicals that have been found to be associated with positive moods include dopamine, serotonin, and oxytocin. For example, oxytocin is associated with feelings of maternal bonding with infants, romantic attachment, and contentment. Researchers continue to study whether oxytocin helps to produce emotions associated with affection, is a by-product of those feelings, or both.[20] Some of these neurotransmitters are also produced during exercise, accounting for the so-called "runner's high" and the association between happiness and physical activity.
- **Our DNA.** As noted previously, research indicates that roughly half of our "average or baseline level of well-being"—our propensity toward cheerfulness or pessimism—is determined by genetics.[21]
- **Our thoughts.** To a significant extent, we are who we perceive ourselves to be. A group of European researchers use the term *positive orientation* to describe how our judgments about ourselves influence our psychological functioning and

well-being. Our levels of life satisfaction, self-esteem, and optimism are guided by how we reflect on life experiences and frame events.[22]

• **Our behaviors.** When scientists today study how our behaviors influence our happiness, they are following a line of inquiry that dates back to Aristotle's teachings that how we interact with others, guided by ethics and virtues such as courage and generosity, is at the core of our well-being.[23] In Chapter 3, we will explore how we can increase our happiness through our actions and interactions with others.

What most of these emotional influences have in common is that we can change them. And by consciously changing our thoughts and behaviors, which has an effect on the production of neurochemicals, we can more consistently achieve positive emotional states. In other words, with the exception of our inherited emotional propensity, we can control most of these influences and over time foster a more positive outlook more of the time in our lives.

Debating the Link Between Money and Happiness

Anyone who has lain awake at night worrying about how to pay the bills knows intuitively that there is a link between money and happiness, especially in terms of alleviating stress and increasing life satisfaction. The debate focuses on whether there is a point beyond which money does not increase happiness. Based on their analysis of data from the Gallup-Healthways Well-Being Index, psychologist Daniel Kahneman and economist Angus Deaton concluded that emotional well-being among Americans increases until annual income reaches $75,000 and then levels off—although life evaluation, "the thoughts that people have about their life," continues to rise steadily with income.[24]

In their analysis of the connection between subjective well-being and income, economists Betsey Stevenson and Justin Wolfers argue for a direct relationship between well-being and income that "does not diminish as income rises. If there is a satiation point, we are yet to reach it."[25] Stevenson and Wolfers suggest that their findings do not conflict with Kahneman and Deaton's conclusions, which they say "are based on very different measures of well-being."

Still, others take issue with the logic of a limitless connection between money and well-being. Seligman, for example, makes the case that people above the "safety net" of income might well value their time more than the opportunity to earn more money. Someone earning $10,000 would leap at the chance for a second job working weekends that would earn an additional $10,000, Seligman reasons, but someone else earning $100,000 might not find that offer so attractive.

Since the mid-20th century, the gross domestic product in the United States has tripled and average income has climbed as well (the Russell Sage Foundation reports that, adjusted for inflation, average family income in the United States rose from $31,886 in 1947 to $82,843 in 2012), but ratings of life satisfaction have not budged and measures of ill-being, such as the incidence of depression and anxiety, have gotten much worse, Seligman notes. His conclusion: "Material prosperity matters ... but only insofar as it increases well-being."[26]

Other researchers have found that what people do with their money influences their emotional well-being. Supporting worthy causes, traveling and taking family vacations, and learning a new skill or hobby are associated with positive emotions much more so than purchasing material goods. "Money increases happiness if it is spent on activities that enhance personal growth or provide new learning experiences—or even if we spend it on small pleasures such as a massage or a long phone call with a friend abroad."[27]

Moving beyond happiness as an emotional state, there is more to maintaining a positive outlook than how we feel from moment to moment. In his book *Authentic Happiness*, Seligman describes three main components of happiness: pleasure, engagement, and meaning.[28] In this model, pleasure represents the "feel-good" part of happiness, the immediate positive emotions we may experience while in the relaxing company of family and friends or when engaged in an entertaining pastime such as playing a game or gardening. Engagement refers to the philosophical concept of pursuing *the good life*, in which we experience the satisfaction of putting our "signature strengths" to use to enrich our existence and the lives of others. Finally, Seligman suggests, we find happiness in making a meaningful contribution to a larger purpose, to our loved ones, to our communities, and even to the greater society. Lyubomirsky offers a similar definition of *happiness* as "the experience of joy, contentment, or positive well-being, combined with a sense that one's life is good, meaningful, and worthwhile."[29]

Seligman expanded his definition of happiness to include five elements of personal well-being, which he calls "the topic of positive psychology," in his book *Flourish*.[30] Those elements are represented by the acronym PERMA:

- **Positive emotion,** as represented by feelings of happiness and satisfaction with life;
- **Engagement,** or the pleasure that comes from being immersed or absorbed by an endeavor;
- **Relationships,** or positive interactions with other people, such as the feelings of well-being that come from helping others;
- **Meaning,** as in finding purpose in your pursuits; and
- **Accomplishment,** or achieving something you value.

The PERMA formulation puts a stronger emphasis on committing our strengths and virtues, such as kindness, social intelligence, humor, courage, and integrity, "to meet the highest challenges that come your way," Seligman writes. "Deploying your highest strengths leads to more positive emotion, to more meaning, to more accomplishment, and to better relationships."[31] To a great extent, then, feeling good is about doing good.

Applying these definitions, we can see that how people experience happiness is highly individual, based on each person's unique blend of heritable traits and dispositions, family background, life experiences, strengths, interests, current outlooks and attitudes, and life goals. Despite these differences, we all have the ability to achieve greater happiness, which in turn can help propel us in positive directions in our personal and professional lives.

Spirituality and Religion as Sources of Happiness

For many people, spirituality or religion provides a deep and abiding source of happiness in terms of fostering positive emotions such as hope, joy, and optimism as well as a sense of meaning, purpose, and overall life satisfaction. The positive effects include fostering virtues such as compassion and self-control and supporting mental and physical health. There is a substantial body of research in the area.[32]

Tapping into the Science of Happiness

The approach to increased happiness, achievement, and wellbeing set out in this book is not just taken from personal experience or some nebulous theory. It is based on research from fields including social cognitive and affective neuroscience and positive psychology. The latter refers to a whole field of applied research that has developed since the late 1990s to study how to help people attain and maintain happiness and reap its many benefits. In their book *Positive Psychology: The Science of Happiness and Flourishing*, William Compton and Edward Hoffman cite the simple but apt definition from the International Positive Psychology Association that "positive psychology is the scientific study of what enables individuals and communities to thrive."[33]

Martin Seligman and Mihalyi Csikszentmihalyi are credited with launching positive psychology in 1998 with the aim of directing scientific scrutiny on the biological, personal, cultural, and other dimensions of positive subjective states and emotions, positive individual traits, and the role of institutions such as employers, schools, and governments in supporting positive human functioning. In a special issue of *American Psychologist* dedicated to positive psychology, Sheldon and King describe its aim to find out "what works, what's right, and what's improving [for] 'the average person.'" They suggest that this still-developing field provides an opportunity for psychologists "to adopt a more open and appreciative perspective regarding human potentials, motives, and capacities" rather than to focus on shortcomings and illness.[34]

Thus, science has joined other avenues of inquiry, including philosophy (e.g., with its examination of philanthropy) and spirituality (e.g., seeking tranquility through meditation), in studying the positive emotional state that so many people strive to attain and that can make a deep and permanent positive difference in their lives. According to the *World Happiness Report*, researchers seeking to study and measure happiness define it both as an emotion ("Were you happy yesterday?") and as an evaluation ("Are you happy with your life as a whole?").[35]

We have incorporated "the science of happiness" in our work in teacher education since the late 1990s. We have long advocated for the importance of positive learning environments, an optimistic approach to learning, and positive relationships among teachers and students: "A fundamental purpose of the BrainSMART approach ... is to help teachers to motivate students to want to learn, to facilitate their learning in a positive and productive learning environment, and to equip them with strategies that support attention, retention, and application of new knowledge and skills."[36] At the core of our books and the curriculum we codeveloped for graduate degree programs for teachers is the message, supported by practical strategies, that an optimistic outlook and positive environment in which students feel safe, secure, accepted, and encouraged to take intellectual risks are crucial for learning success. We share some of those strategies throughout this book.

Before the dawn of positive psychology, many scientists dismissed the idea of studying what they considered to be a nebulous, even trivial, subject. The investigation of emotions was channeled toward correcting ills such as the diagnosis and treatment of depression and the study of criminal behavior rooted in anger and despair. Near the dawn of psychology in the late nineteenth and early twentieth centuries, the pioneers of this new field shied away from emotions, "considered too slippery to be legitimate targets of study," Fredrickson notes, and when psychologists did begin to study emotions, they focused on "depression, aggression, anxiety, and all the ills that negative states like these can produce in people's lives."[37] Lyubomirsky suggests that this fixation on "disease, disorder, and the negative side of life" persisted into the mid- and late 20th century.[38] Compton and Hoffman contrast this traditional paradigm with the new path offered by positive psychology:

> All too often psychological research has displayed a blatant bias toward assumptions that people are unwitting pawns of their biology, their childhood, and their unconscious. Previous psychological theories have often argued that human beings are determined by their past; by their biology, their cultural conditioning and unconscious motives. Positive psychology takes the position that despite the very real difficulties of life, it must be acknowledged that most people adjust quite well to life's ups and downs.[39]

The aim of the longstanding focus of psychology was to alleviate depression, anger, and aggression, with the assumption that a reduction in these negative states would result in an increase in positive emotions. Unfortunately, when people go to therapy in order to rid themselves of psychological problems, they don't necessarily become happier. Lessening depression doesn't leave a vacuum that is automatically filled with a positive outlook. As Seligman puts it, "positive mental health is not just the absence of mental illness. ... Positive mental health is a presence, the presence of engagement, the presence of meaning, the presence of good relationships, and the presence of accomplishment."[40] Each of us has the capacity to learn to think intentionally in ways that will make us happier and more likely to achieve the goals we set for ourselves.

The still-emerging field of positive psychology approaches the challenge of how to nurture personal well-being from this opposing perspective. In the course of their work, psychologists like Seligman, Lyubomirsky, and Fredrickson have come to recognize that positive emotional states can help alleviate some significant problems. A lack of well-being has been shown to be a precursor in the onset of depression, and forms of therapy that focus on helping people develop more positive emotions in their lives have proven to be as effective as older forms that aimed to reduce negative emotions. With this progression in understanding has come an increasing emphasis on studying positive emotions in their own right, not just as an antidote for depression.

Achieving Greater Happiness Through Practical Metacognition

At the core of positive psychology is another fundamental finding: Not only can happiness make our lives better, we can make ourselves happier—and thus enjoy more of the benefits that come from this positive state of being. One of several deep-seated misconceptions we will bring to the surface with the aim of eradicating it is that people's outlooks and attitudes are largely fixed and unchangeable. According to this persistent but mistaken belief, a predilection toward optimism or pessimism is our birthright and defines how we think about opportunities and our likelihood of succeeding in achieving the goals we set for ourselves throughout life.

To the contrary, our genetic makeup, family background, and life experiences account for only part of our outlook on life and our ability to experience and sustain joy. As Lyubomirsky suggests, we all have "opportunities to increase or decrease our happiness levels through what we do in our daily lives and how we think."[41]

Throughout these pages, we will explore how happiness and success in achieving our personal and professional goals are inextricably intertwined, how more of one produces more of the other, and how we can consciously optimize this dynamic in a continual upward spiral. Research at the foundation of positive psychology concludes that "while being successful can make one feel happier, the converse is also true: being happier can lead to greater success later in life! By helping people both to reach their potential and to eliminate negative emotions and problematic behaviors, the study of positive emotions and adaptive behavior can thereby offer beneficiaries more fulfilling lives."[42]

In short, happiness can lead us to become what we describe as "positively smarter." We define *smart* as being able to learn new ideas and skills, to solve problems, to work productively with others, to come up with creative ideas, and to share our ideas through effective communication. Developing and applying a positive outlook can help us to improve in these endeavors—to get progressively smarter.

Cognition refers to the thinking processes at work as you acquire knowledge and develop new skills. Thinking about your thinking with the goal of improving those cognitive processes—to get positively smarter—is called *metacognition*. A wide body of educational research supports the academic gains across all subjects that are possible when students are taught how and when to use cognitive and metacognitive strategies to take charge of their learning. The same is true for adults: Through the use of what we call *practical metacognition*, which will be explored in Chapter 5, you can make steady progress in developing the skills and knowledge necessary to accomplish your goals. The CIA Model (for control, influence, and acknowledge) offers a useful and versatile example of practical metacognition.

Applying the CIA Model

To make the most of the power of neuroplasticity to become positively smarter requires that we invest our time, energy, and thinking wisely. The mind tends to be drawn to negative topics and events almost like the pull of gravity, as research discussed in Chapter 3 will show. Particularly unproductive is the tendency to gravitate toward negatives over which we have no control or minimal influence. The solution, as represented in this model, is to take a step back and focus first on what we can **control** through our thoughts and actions and where we can have a positive **influence** on the results we want to produce. We also need to briefly **acknowledge** those areas that are beyond our control and influence. Then we can choose where to invest our attention and energies for the best possible outcomes.

Control　Channel your thoughts, time, effort, and energy on what provides the greatest positive payoff to achieve your goals and to balance all the important components of your life—family and friends, work, physical and emotional health, and personal pursuits. Understand and take charge of what is within your control: your attitudes and mindfulness, gratitude for and appreciation of that which brings pleasure, development and improvement of knowledge and skills, responsibility for healthy nutrition and exercise, completion of important tasks at work and at home, time spent with family and friends, and participation in your community.

Influence　Recognize the factors that influence your thinking and actions, including your beliefs and knowledge and the beliefs and expectations of influential people in your life. Some influences may persist below your level of awareness unless you apply a metacognitive approach to ferret them out, and they may even be counterproductive to your goal of becoming positively smarter. Focus on thoughts and actions that can have the most positive impact in areas and situations where you have some influence, in your own life, happiness, and sense of satisfaction and in supporting others by listening, encouraging, praising, giving useful feedback, and pitching in to collaborate and get the work done.

Acknowledge Acknowledge that there are people and situations where you have little or no influence. Spending time fretting and complaining about these areas is a waste of valuable time and energy. In studying discord in marriages, for example, John Gottman and Julie Schwartz Gottman discovered that many arguments are never resolved but fester and persist to the point of sometimes shattering relationships.[43] This is an example of where acknowledging that we need to agree to disagree can be helpful.

Let's explore how we might apply this approach in the domain of happiness.

CIA in Action: Happiness and Subjective Well-Being

"There is only one way to happiness and that is to cease worrying about things which are beyond the power of our will."

—Epictetus

Control: Focus on the factors that account for some 40 percent of happiness, and implement practical strategies that research suggests can increase levels of optimism and happiness, such as those presented in Chapter 3.

Influence: Your personal level of optimistic thinking, happiness, and overall life satisfaction and the impact you can have by maintaining positive relationships with family, friends, coworkers, and others in your life.

Acknowledge: That part of your happiness is driven by genetic predisposition and that you have little control over negative situations and people who prefer to focus on pessimism and negativity. Minimize time and energy expended on these factors where you have limited control and influence.

Notes

1 William C. Compton and Edward Hoffman. 2013. *Positive Psychology: The Science of Happiness and Flourishing* (2nd ed.). Belmont, CA: Wadsworth, p. 51.

2 Wadi Rum Films. *Happy* (PBS Special), 2012.

3 John Helliwell, Richard Layard, and Jeffrey Sachs, Editors. *World Happiness Report 2013*. New York: United Nations. Retrieved from http://unsdsn. org/wp-content/uploads/2014/02/WorldHappinessReport2013_online.pdf

4 Richard J. Davidson, with Sharon Begley. 2012. *The Emotional Life of Your Brain*. New York: Hudson Street Press, p. 89.

5 Barbara Fredrickson. 2009. *Positivity: Groundbreaking Research Reveals How to Embrace the Hidden Strength of Positive Emotions, Overcome Negativity, and Thrive*. New York: Crown, p. 21.

6 Mark Batey. "Creativity Is the Key Skill for the 21st Century." *The Creativity Post*, March 28, 2012. Retrieved from http://www.creativitypost. com/business/creativity_is_the_key_skill_for_the_21st_century#sthash.8h6pm Amq.dpuf

7 Martin E. P. Seligman. 2011. *Flourish: A Visionary New Understanding of Happiness and Well-Being*. New York: Crown, p. 22.

8 Seligman, *Flourish*, p. 20.

9 Jessica Pryce-Jones. "Ways to Be Happy and Productive at Work." *The Wall Street Journal*, November 25, 2012. Retrieved from http://blogs. wsj.com/source/2012/11/25/five-ways-to-be-happy-and-productive-at-work/

10 Andrew J. Oswald, Eugenio Proto, and Daniel Sgroi. *Happiness and Productivity* (3rd version). Retrieved from http://www2.warwick.ac.uk/ fac/soc/economics/staff/eproto/workingpapers/happinessproductivity.pdf

11 Peter Schulman. "Applying 'Learned Optimism' to Increase Sales Productivity." *Journal of Personal Selling and Sales Management*, *19*(1), Winter 1999, 31. Retrieved from http://www.waldentesting.com/ salestests/sasq/SASQ%20article.PDF

12 Noomii. "Happiness & Career Success" [Infographic]. *The Un-Self-Help Blog*, September 18, 2013. Retrieved from http://www.noomii.com/ blog/5104-happiness-career-success-infographic

13 Seligman, *Flourish*, pp. 205–207.

14 Viktor Frankl. 1946/1984. *Man's Search for Meaning* (Ilse Lasch, trans.). New York: Washington Square Press.

15 Fredrickson, p. 99.

16 Teresa Aubele and Susan Reynolds. "Happy Brain, Happy Life." *Prime Your Gray Cells* (Psychology Today blog), August 2, 2011. Retrieved from http://www.psychologytoday.com/blog/prime-your-gray-cells/201108/happy-brain-happy-life

17 Sonja Lyubomirsky, Laura King, and Ed Diener. "The Benefits of Frequent Positive Affect: Does Happiness Lead to Success?" *Psychological Bulletin*, *131*(6), 2005, p. 840.

18 Sonja Lyubomirsky. 2007. *The How of Happiness: A New Approach to Getting the Life You Want*. New York: Penguin, pp. 20–21.

19 Lyubomirsky, p. 22.

20 Davidson, p. 74.

21 Compton and Hoffman, pp. 26–27.

22 Gian Vittorio Caprara. "Positive Orientation: Turning Potentials into Optimal Functioning." *The European Health Psychologist, 11,* September 2009. Retrieved from http://openhealthpsychology.net/ehp/issues/2009/v11iss3_Sept2009/EHP_Sept09_Caprara.pdf; G. V. Caprara, P. Steca, G. Alessandri, J. R. Abela, and C. M. McWhinnie. "Positive Orientation: Explorations on What Is Common to Life Satisfaction, Self-Esteem, and Optimism." *Epidemiology and Psychiatric Sciences, 19*(1), January–March 2010, 63–71.

23 Compton and Hoffman, p. 29.

24 Daniel Kahneman and Angus P. Deaton. "High Income Improves Evaluation of Life But Not Emotional Well-Being." *Proceedings of the National Academy of Sciences of the United States of America, 107*(38), September 21, 2010. Retrieved from http://www.pnas.org/content/107/38/16489.full

25 Betsey Stevenson and Justin Wolfers. "Subjective Well-Being and Income: Is There Any Evidence of Satiation?" *American Economic Review, Papers and Proceedings,* May 2013.

26 Seligman, *Flourish,* p. 221.

27 Compton and Hoffman, p. 64.

28 Martin Seligman. 2002. *Authentic Happiness: Using the New Positive Psychology to Realize Your Potential for Lasting Fulfillment.* New York: Simon & Schuster.

29 Lyubomirsky, p. 32.

30 Seligman, *Flourish,* p. 24.

31 Ibid.

32 Compton and Hoffman, pp. 229–230.

33 Compton and Hoffman, p. 2.

34 Kennon Sheldon and Laura King. "Why Positive Psychology Is Necessary." *American Psychologist, 54*(3), March 2001, p. 216.

35 Helliwell, Layard, and Sachs, p. 3.

36 Donna Wilson and Marcus Conyers. 2011. *BrainSMART 60 Strategies for Increasing Student Learning* (4th ed.). Orlando, FL: BrainSMART, p. 23.

37 Fredrickson, p. 12.

38 Lyubomirsky, p. 3.

39 Compton and Hoffman, p. 5.

40 Seligman, *Flourish,* p. 183.

41 Lyubomirsky, p. 22.

42 Compton and Hoffman, p. 5.

43 John M. Gottman and Julie Schwartz Gottman. 2006. *10 Lessons to Transform Your Marriage.* New York: Crown.

3

Stop Daydreaming and Start Thinking Your Way to Higher Levels of Happiness
Focused Fifteen Strategies for Boosting Positivity

"Happiness is best regarded as a skill. . . . We can actually take responsibility for our minds and brains and cultivate healthy habits of mind. Through that, we can change our brains in ways that promote well-being."
—Richard J. Davidson[1]

Studying happiness in people's daily lives can be challenging. It's not like researchers can follow their subjects around, measuring their emotional responses as they work, play, spend time with their families, and carry out their everyday routines. How might scientists stay in touch with the people they are studying?

Via their mobile phones, of course.

Harvard researchers Matthew Killingsworth and Daniel Gilbert developed an iPhone app to gather data from a broad range of volunteers "at random moments during their waking hours,"[2] to pinpoint how they were feeling, what they were doing, and what they were thinking about. This medium of research and these questions permitted the researchers to check in with volunteer respondents in the midst of their everyday tasks and to find out how they were feeling as they were daydreaming—to test a common assumption that minds wander away from routine tasks in search of more

Positively Smarter: Science and Strategies for Increasing Happiness, Achievement, and Well-Being, First Edition. Marcus Conyers and Donna Wilson.

pleasant things to ponder. According to this line of thought, daydreaming would be a way to insert more happiness into humdrum activities.

Analyzing nearly 250,000 responses from 5,000 participants in 83 countries across a wide range of ages and occupations, the researchers reported three findings, some of which you might find unexpected: (1) in almost half of the situations recorded, people's thoughts were not on the activities they were currently undertaking; (2) "people were less happy when their minds were wandering than when they were not";[3] and (3) people's thoughts were a better predictor of their level of happiness than their actions in the moment.

These findings support a key big idea that happiness can best be found by being present in the moment, not by daydreaming, longing to be elsewhere, or worrying about the past or future. In effect, the study suggests that "a wandering mind is an unhappy mind." The conclusion that our unfocused minds steer us away from happiness may seem surprising at first. After all, don't we daydream out of boredom or to imagine ourselves in a happier place? The problem is that, without direction, our minds gravitate to negative thoughts; as Seligman notes, "we think too much about what goes wrong and not enough about what goes right in our lives."[4] It takes conscious effort to focus on the positive and, in doing so, to create and maintain a consistently brighter outlook.

In a sense, focus is the fulcrum of happiness, the pivot point you can position to amplify your positive perspective and enhance your productivity and well-being. As the research presented in Chapter 1 points out—and as the quote that opens this chapter reinforces—over time you have the power to choose your attitude, to decide to achieve higher levels of happiness more of the time, and to work toward that goal by cultivating attitudes and skills that support a positive outlook. In this chapter, we present the "Focused Fifteen," strategies and skills you can develop to channel your wandering mind with the aim of becoming happier and more successful in achieving your personal and professional goals.

Table 3.1 Action Assessment: Focusing on a Positive Outlook

Before we introduce the Focused Fifteen strategies, complete this chart to establish your baseline of "happiness know-how." Are these actions currently part of your daily life? (We will revisit this assessment at the end of the book.)

On a daily basis, how often do you ...	Almost never	Sometimes	Frequently	Consistently
1. Savor the wow of now.				
2. Work at consciously maintaining an upbeat attitude.				
3. Picture a positive future.				
4. Actively commit acts of kindness.				
5. Acknowledge and appreciate the good things in your life.				
6. Recognize and set aside negative thoughts and worries.				
7. Take time to relate to others in positive ways.				
8. Achieve a state of flow or find yourself "in the zone."				
9. Set and monitor your progress toward positive goals.				
10. Respond with resilience to tough challenges.				

(continued)

Table 3.1 Action Assessment: Focusing on a Positive Outlook (*cont'd*)

On a daily basis, how often do you ...	*Almost never*	*Sometimes*	*Frequently*	*Consistently*
11. Look past others' real and imagined transgressions to let go of anger and resentment.				
12. Move your body to boost your mood.				
13. Smile frequently and naturally.				
14. Play to your peak strengths.				
15. Identify and share the treasures in your life.				

Connecting Thinking and Feeling

Intellect and emotions have traditionally been viewed as separate spheres. People tended to think of emotions as illogical and likely to cloud thinking and reasoning. In popular culture, this dichotomy might be best represented in the *Star Trek* characters of Spock and Dr. McCoy. Today, however, we know that thinking and feeling are inextricably interwoven. A positive emotional state and optimistic outlook facilitate learning; conversely, thoughts can influence and help direct feelings. According to psychology professor Richard Davidson, "Emotion works with cognition in an integrated and seamless way to enable us to navigate the world of relationships, work, and spiritual growth."[5] Perhaps in reflection of this new understanding of the connection between thinking and feeling, the Spock in the latest *Star Trek* reboot is permitted to demonstrate affection, loyalty, and other very human emotions!

As the title of this book implies, becoming positively smarter entails concerted effort to enhance both your emotional outlook and cognitive abilities, and one influences the other. You can think your way to a happier you, and a more positive approach to life can increase your motivation and commitment to develop new skills and abilities.

Becoming smarter is not just about increasing your intellect. Rather than taking a narrow view of intelligence, we ascribe to a wider perspective on the range of cognitive capabilities people can develop to thrive in their personal and work lives, including practical problem-solving skills, creativity and an innovative mindset, and interpersonal and communication abilities.[6] Emotional intelligence is another crucial form of intellectual development that brings together thinking and feeling. Emotional intelligence, or EQ, "is the foundation for a host of critical skills—it impacts most everything you say and do each day. ... It's the single biggest predictor of performance in the workplace and the strongest driver of leadership and personal excellence."[7] EQ, which is characterized by the ability to recognize and manage one's emotions and to interact productively with others, has been identified as the "secret weapon" that allows people with average IQs to outperform those with high IQs 70 percent of the time.[8] There's even an app for developing your EQ, from the Yale Center for Emotional Intelligence. The App Mood Meter (see MoodMeter-App.com) provides a means for recognizing and regulating your affective states. It might work well in evaluating the impact of some of the strategies presented in this chapter on enhancing your positivity.

Practical metacognition (see Chapter 5) provides a pathway to enhance your emotional and other forms of intelligence and to nurture a more consistently positive and productive outlook. Over time, monitoring your thoughts and feelings to keep them focused in a purposeful and positive direction will result in steady progress toward these intertwined aims. Guiding your thinking to maintain an optimistic approach "changes the scope or boundaries of your mind [and] widens the span of possibilities that you see."[9] By changing the way you think, you can change the way you feel. In effect, you can think your way to greater levels of happiness!

The "workhorse" of practical metacognition to make the most of this juncture of emotion and cognition is selective attention, the ability to direct your mind from wandering into negative thoughts and worries and to stay focused on the positive. By developing your selective attention, you will be able to concentrate on what is important in a given endeavor and attend to what is necessary to accomplish your goals. This is sometimes referred to as "being mindful." Mindfulness training has been demonstrated to improve people's ability to focus their attention on their studies and other important tasks.[10] In terms of the importance of improving one's selective attention, Csikszentmihalyi notes that

> Innate talents cannot develop into a mature intelligence unless a person learns to control attention. Only through extensive investments of psychic energy can a child with musical gifts turn into a musician, or a mathematically gifted child into an engineer or physicist. It takes much effort to absorb the knowledge and the skills that are needed to do the mental operations an adult professional is supposed to perform. Mozart was a prodigy and a genius, but if his father hadn't forced him to practice as soon as he was out of diapers, it is doubtful his talent would have blossomed as it did. By learning to concentrate, a person acquires control over psychic energy, the basic fuel upon which all thinking depends.[11]

You can learn to develop and sharpen your selective attention. When you notice that your mind is wandering toward negative or pessimistic thoughts, ask yourself the WIN question to guide yourself back toward a positive mindset: What's Important Now? Answering this question can help you establish your clear intent to accomplish your goals while maintaining optimism about your likelihood of succeeding. WIN is an acronym to remind you of these important questions:

- **What** do I need to attend to so that I can actualize my clear intent in this situation and stay focused on positive progress?
- What must I choose to **Ignore** so that I can keep moving forward?
- To what do I need to attend to **Now** to create win-win situations and further progress toward my goals?

The payoff for developing selective attention is the ability to stay focused on the most important task or idea of the moment—and to maintain a positive outlook while doing so. In the busy lives many of us lead, the concept of multitasking holds great allure. We believe we can get a lot more done if we do two or three or four things simultaneously. The reality is that our consciousness can have one experience or focus on one thought at a time. We can shift from thought to thought or from task to task quickly, but our brains are not designed to handle two tasks simultaneously, especially when those tasks are similar.[12] If you're listening to the radio and someone starts to talk to you, your brain tunes out the radio to hear what the person is saying. The same goes for surfing the Internet while chatting on the phone with a friend. If something catches your attention online, you will likely miss what your friend is saying while your brain reads and interprets the information on the screen.

Try this experiment to see how these findings apply to maintaining a positive outlook: Think about a joyful event and a boring event at the same time. It's really difficult, isn't it? When you focus on picturing a positive outcome in your mind, you feel good. When you let your mind wander into worrying about a negative outcome, you feel bad. By developing your selective attention, you get to choose.

At any given moment, a person can focus on only a limited number of experiences, positive or negative. We call this *cognitive space*, which is related to the concept of working memory. Vying for attention in our cognitive space is the here and now of our external environment—what we can see, hear, and sense around us—and our internal focus, or lack thereof. Cognitive space is limited and valuable. Selective attention helps make the most of it.

We are not suggesting that all daydreaming is bad. In fact, "freeing your mind" and letting it wander away from a perplexing problem is often the path to creative solutions.[13] However, monitoring when your thoughts drift into negative territory and purposefully steering your attention back to a more positive outlook can help make happiness a habit—and get you to solutions to those puzzling dilemmas quicker!

The Focused Fifteen

Happiness researchers have found that actually applying simple strategies similar to our following favorites can help people boost their positive outlook, take a more optimistic approach to much of what they do, and become more resilient when confronted with obstacles. So far in this book we have shared a great deal of research from psychology, neuroscience, and education. We take a more light-hearted approach in sharing the following strategies to make them more memorable and "sticky" for you. You might want to start with one and over time introduce additional strategies to find which ones work best for you.

1. Savor the Wow of Now

Find "oceanic" moments in every day.

In our busy everyday lives, it is easy to forget to stop and take time to savor what can be great sources of joy. A useful habit to cultivate is to notice and appreciate people, places, and activities in your daily life with which you have happy associations, even if only for a few minutes. Turn off the "background noise" of worries and deadlines and focus on a pleasant conversation with your spouse or children. Enjoy lunch with a friend. Pay attention to the scenery along your favorite walking path—and try new routes for a change of pace. Watch a sunset or sunrise. Engage in a favorite hobby or pastime.

Savoring the wow of now is about focusing on the UPside, associated with being:

- **Useful,** in moving toward accomplishing your goals, completing tasks, and solving problems, and/or
- **Positive,** in spending time with people, in places, and in activities that are enjoyable in their own right and make you feel happy, refreshed, and rejuvenated.

Think of the things you can focus on in your daily environment along a continuum that ranges from Relaxed Positive (fun) and Useful Positive (energized at work) to Useless Negative (hanging on to emotions that serve little purpose other than making you feel bad). In the middle of this continuum are neutral activities that have little emotional impact and what we call Useful Negatives, tasks and activities that may seem frustrating and irritating but ultimately lead to progress and a path to more positive states. Like the App Mood Meter mentioned previously, this continuum sets out in a concrete way the emotions you may experience on a daily basis so that you can more purposefully aim to maintain a positive outlook.

Relaxed Positive	Laughing with a friend, playing a game or reading a beloved book with the kids, going to a concert or ballgame, watching the sunset
Useful Positive	In the flow with a work project, training for a race, or learning a new language
Useful Neutral	Paying the bills, cleaning the house, weeding the garden
Useful Negative	Feeling overwhelmed and confused at the start of a work project, but staying resolved to develop a plan and learn the necessary new skills to tackle it; engaging in deliberate practice to get better at a necessary subskill
Useless Negative	Whining, complaining, and obsessing over mistakes and slights

By savoring the wow of now, you can spend more time at the top of this continuum, be as productive as possible in the middle, and avoid the bottom more often!

Donna shares her own example of savoring the wow of now: Marcus and I were out for a morning bike ride. I was feeling a little conflicted about taking time out from work, feeling the pressure of deadlines, and my leg muscles were burning a bit from peddling through the sand. But then I looked up as the sun broke through the clouds. I saw diamonds glinting in the deep turquoise of the gulf waters and the crystal sands of the beach, heard the crash of waves and calls of gulls, and took in the fresh scent of the sea. It was such a perfect moment that I laughed out loud. We use the term "oceanic" to capture that feeling of tranquility and transformation in finding such beauty in our surroundings—wherever we are. We now seek out oceanic moments when we are traveling and hiking up a mountain, strolling through the countryside, taking in the sights, sounds, and smells at a farmers' market, or finding ourselves captivated at a concert or art gallery. You might have your own terms to describe those perfect moments that transform and reenergize—"huggable," "shooting the rapids," "crossing the finish line," "fit of laughter," "purr-fect." Wherever you find bliss is worth revisiting and capturing in your memory for easy retrieval.

2. Work at Maintaining an Upbeat Attitude with Positive Self-Talk

Purposefully shift from self-nagging to pay yourself a compliment when you've earned one.

Our inner feelings and thoughts influence how we feel about and interact with others and the world around us, so we must focus on developing positive self-talk and self-image that will then radiate outward. Consider these two examples of inner monologue as the day begins:

Sam: I HATE THAT ALARM! I don't want to get up. And I DEFINITELY don't want to go to work today. ... Late already. Can't find my keys. … Stuck in a traffic jam, where that stupid thing I said yesterday at work just replays in my mind. Over and over and over again. Now I'm never going to get that promotion. I am such an idiot.

Mel: Glad I switched radio stations on my alarm. Much more pleasant to wake up to classical music. … Yum, love the smell of this new coffee! And glad I've gotten into the habit of stacking my work stuff and keys on the counter so I can find everything when it's time to go. … Another traffic jam, but at least I can think through how I can clarify what I said in the meeting yesterday. Not my best presentation, for sure. I could see that my boss was a little confused. … Oh, wait, I think if I back up a little and provide some more details, that should paint a clearer picture of our proposal. Maybe even a diagram. That helped a lot for the last project. Hmm …

Both of these examples include the same challenges: having to get up and out to work on time, dealing with the daily traffic, and pondering how to recover from a misstep at work. The first person wakes up feeling discontented, and the day gets worse from there. Instead of dealing with minor annoyances like a loud alarm and lost keys, Sam moans and complains. Stuck in a traffic jam, Sam increases the volume on negative self-talk and self-doubt, expecting the worst at work rather than pondering solutions. Mel, on the other hand, wakes up appreciating a softer alarm, fresh coffee, and a plan he has put in place to have the keys and other necessities ready to roll. A traffic jam is no fun, but Mel uses the time to brainstorm ways to recover from a poor presentation. Rather than catastrophizing the setback, he focuses on recovery and moving forward.

Based on his work on learned optimism and the power of a positive outlook, Martin Seligman has suggested that people essentially learn their thinking through a set of questions when something goes right or wrong.[14] Table 3.2 applies those questions to Sam and Mel's perspectives.

Table 3.2 Positive vs. Negative Self-Talk

Question that relates to outlook:	Translation:	Answer from Sam's point of view:	How Mel might respond:
Is it personal?	Is it really up to me?	"Every morning is a hassle. That annoying alarm and rushing around to get ready, only to get stuck in a traffic jam!"	"My new alarm, that yummy coffee, and my plan to get organized the night before makes the morning a lot easier. And I can't end the traffic jam, but I do appreciate the think time!"
Is it pervasive?	Does it affect every part of my life?	"A frantic morning sets the stage for a miserable day at work, especially because I have to face everyone after screwing up at the meeting yesterday."	"When I have a hard time at work, I do my best to leave it at work. After a good run and time to relax in the evening, I can deal with work problems with a fresh perspective the next day."
Is it permanent?	Will it be here forever? Can it be changed?	"Now I'll never get that promotion!"	"I've got a plan to follow up on the presentation that should set us on the right track!"

When something goes wrong, optimists are likely to fix what is within their control and recognize what is not. They are good at depersonalizing and compartmentalizing setbacks at work so they don't spill over into their personal lives (and vice versa). And they treat minor, temporary setbacks for what they are instead of blowing them out of proportion. In comparison, pessimists have a far different reaction: "It's all my fault. It's going to ruin every part of my life. And it's never going to get better." These responses have a neurological component: Greater activation in the brain's left hemisphere is associated with optimism, a sense of control over one's ability to effect positive change, and persistent effort to do so, while the right hemisphere is more active when people are feeling pessimistic, fearful, and powerless. In keeping with the primary assertion of this chapter, brain research also shows "conscious and mindful effort" to focus on the positive can help increase left-hemispheric activation and reinforce an optimistic outlook.[15]

By training ourselves to answer these questions in more productive ways, Seligman suggests that we can adopt and maintain a more positive outlook. Try these ideas to shift your negative self-talk to positive reinforcement:

- When you feel your mind wandering into negative thoughts, worries, and complaints, purposefully steer your thinking in a more optimistic direction. Picture positive outcomes. Call to mind a person or memory that always makes you smile.
- When you run into an obstacle or setback, take a step back and consider the possible solutions and upsides in the situation. Complaining is easy; finding positive take-aways requires digging a bit deeper and learning from the experience. Sharing a personal example, we worked hard for three months on a proposal for a project that did not materialize. Rather than just letting that work go to waste, we stepped back, looked at it with fresh eyes, and created two different projects—for which we landed contracts—that were even more on target!
- When you feel down about yourself or your abilities, focus on your positive qualities. Give yourself a compliment. It needn't

be flowery and overblown. In fact, it should be authentic, and it may be relatively simple: "I am really good at organizing things." "I am a good friend because I listen well." "I am persistent in sticking with a task until I get it done."

Incorporating positive self-talk into your daily life will improve your overall mood and ability to respond to challenging situations. You may find opportunities to apply it in your interactions with family and friends. Donna recalls difficult conversations with a dear friend who had lost her husband several years ago: Whenever we talked on the phone, she was quite withdrawn. I knew she appreciated hearing from me, but it was so hard to draw her into talking about anything positive—or even talking much at all. After overhearing one of those conversations, Marcus later said, "I hate to hear you go through the distress of this lack of connection. You are trying so hard, and she is so distant." He reminded me that both of us enjoy flowers and gardening and suggested that this might be a good topic to engage her. From that day forward, most times when we talk, we have pleasant conversations about her garden. What a difference emphasizing the positive makes in terms of the outcome! It doesn't mean that every interaction we have is all sweetness and light or that all we talk about is flowers. If she wants to talk about missing her husband, that's what we talk about. The important thing is that we are talking, and it is good to hear the happiness in her voice when she describes her garden and shares her plans for planting new flowers.

3. Picture a Positive Future

Viktor Frankl provides an inspiring example of taking responsibility for one's attitude even in extremely difficult circumstances.

A dramatic example of the power of a positive outlook comes from Viktor Frankl's memoir of surviving the horrors of an Auschwitz concentration camp by "living for the future." In his classic book *Man's Search for Meaning,* Frankl vividly recalls how he rose above feeling hunger, cold, and severe pain and being surrounded by despair by picturing himself in the future standing on the platform of a warm amphitheater lecturing about his philosophy of surviving and thriving. Though they were prisoners in the most dire circumstances, Frankl writes that he and his comrades held on to "the last of the human freedoms—to choose one's attitude in any given circumstances, to choose one's own way."[16]

To make the positive future you envision for yourself and those you love as concrete as possible, visualize it and capture it in a journal where you can set out your future goals in writing, enumerate the incremental steps to achieve those goals, and track your progress. Include diagrams, pictures, even doodles about the bright future you envision and the positive steps you are taking in that direction.

4. Kindness the Killer App

Kindness often kindles a positive chain reaction.

Our own happiness benefits from the kindness we extend to others. Extensive research around the world enumerates a variety of personal benefits that come from helping others: Kindness results in an immediate boost in happiness, and making it a habit has a long-term positive impact on our emotional well-being.[17] In one such study in the United Kingdom, 86 participants took a survey assessing their life satisfaction and then were divided into three groups. Participants in one group were asked to perform an act of kindness daily for the next 10 days, and the people in another group were asked to try something new every day over the same period. The third group received no instructions. After the trial period, the participants completed the life satisfaction survey again. People in the first two groups reported greater happiness while the control group showed no change. Writing for the website Greater Good: The Science of a Meaningful Life, Alex Dixon also reports on similar research:

> In this study, the researchers instructed roughly half of the 51 participants to recall, as vividly as they could, the last time they spent $20 or $100 on themselves. The other participants had to recall

the last time they spent the same amounts on someone else. All the participants also completed a scale that measured how happy they were.

Researchers then gave the participants small sums of money and two basic choices: They could spend it on themselves (by covering a bill, another expense, or a gift for themselves) or on someone else (through a donation to charity or a gift). Choose whatever will make you happiest, the researchers told them, adding that their choice would remain anonymous, just in case they felt pressure to appear more altruistic.

The researchers made two big findings. First, consistent with the British study, people in general felt happier when they were asked to remember a time they bought something for someone else—even happier than when they remembered buying something for themselves. This happiness boost was the same regardless of whether the gift cost $20 or $100.

But the second finding is even more provocative: The happier participants felt about their past generosity, the more likely they were in the present to choose to spend on someone else instead of themselves. Not all participants who remembered their past kindness felt happy. But the ones who did feel happy were overwhelmingly more likely to double down on altruism.

The results suggest a kind of "positive feedback loop" between kindness and happiness, according to the authors, so that one encourages the other.[18]

Committing acts of kindness increases empathy, decreases stress levels, and has even been shown to lead to longer lives.[19] The benefits of helping one person often reverberate, as that person commits an act of kindness to another, and that person to another, and so on in a positive chain reaction.

You will see these benefits in your own life by staying on alert for opportunities to incorporate random acts of kindness into your daily routine: Commit at least three small acts of kindness and generosity every day, and take note of how you feel after each one. Share vegetables from your garden with your coworkers. Deliver an elderly neighbor's mail to her door on a rainy day. Volunteer at the library or food pantry. Seligman shares a story about distributing free penny stamps at his post office after the cost of stamps went up.[20] A small investment of your time and/or money reaps rewards for both the recipients of your kindness and for your own feelings of well-being.

5. *Active Appreciation: Create and Tune into Your Appreciation Station*

When we actively appreciate all that we have right now, all that we have appreciates.

When we actively appreciate what we have and are authentically grateful for what matters most to us—our family and friends, our health, our work—we can increase our level of happiness in a fundamental way. This appreciation can and should be shared: Thanking people who have made a beneficial difference in our lives produces uplifting emotional responses that in turn "create positive connections among people and allow us to express our highest values and potential."[21] Appreciating the people in our lives helps us stay focused on their best attributes and thus strengthens our relationships. When we actively appreciate all that we have right now, all that we have appreciates.

Appreciation can also be part of your internal dialogue to help maintain a positive outlook. Think of this strategy as programming your own Appreciation Station. Just as you keep the car radio tuned to your favorite station and download your personal "Top 40" songs onto a playlist, you can add to your journal (see strategy 3) to list all that you are grateful for and appreciate in your life. Then make a conscious effort to tune into your Appreciation Station at least once a day to reflect on the good things in your life. You might make this part of your morning or evening routine or incorporate it into transitions during your day. Marcus tunes into his Appreciation Station when he runs. He runs a mile and then pauses to take a deep breath and reflect on some of the people and aspects of his life that he most appreciates.

6. *Give It a Break: Hang Your Problems Away for a While*

Focus on What's Important Now. Your problems can wait.

We don't mean to suggest that a focus on developing a more positive outlook will make your life perfect. Life is full of little problems and occasional big ones. A positive, persistent approach may help you resolve some of these issues, but others may be beyond your control. Have you ever had a persistent problem that nagged at your thoughts and distracted you from your work and personal interactions? It can be difficult not to dwell on this problem and let the resulting negative feelings take charge. But you can choose to consciously set these problems aside for a while using the Coat Hanger Strategy:

- Identify the problem that is distracting you from the activity at hand.
- Consider: Do I have control over this problem? Are there steps I can take right now to resolve or alleviate it?
- If the answer to both questions is "no," imagine draping the problem on a coat hanger and leaving it outside your door so you can return to your current activities without distractions.

Marcus came up with this strategy several years ago while traveling in Canada for business: I'd received a phone call about an illness in the family. I was concerned for my loved one, who was more than 1,000 miles away, and even though I understood there was nothing I could or should do about the problem immediately, I was upset and distracted—and worried that these feelings might keep me from doing the best possible job on the workshop I was presenting for firefighters. So, I came up with an idea: I visualized hanging my worries on a coat hanger outside the room where I would be doing the presentation and then walked through the door to greet the workshop participants. The workshop went well because I was able to focus exclusively on the needs of my audience, and several firefighters stepped up to say they'd learned a lot to help them in their work. I didn't have to feel guilty or worry that I was trying to "forget" about my loved one. In fact, when I needed to be with my family, I was there—and fully in that moment.

I learned a good lesson that day: Our lives are made up of important people and pursuits—some matter more to us than others, of course, but each of them requires us at some point to put aside other concerns and focus on What's Important Now (remember the WIN question?). When we are with friends and family, they deserve our full attention. When we are working on a big project, we can do a much better job if we focus on it. And we can find joy in our personal pursuits—a long run, a bountiful garden, an engine rebuilt—if we allow ourselves to be immersed and in flow. We've shared this strategy with thousands of people attending our workshops, and many report back that they have found it to be a useful way to choose where to focus their attention to optimize their time spent on any endeavor.

7. Treat Your Relationships Like a Treasure (Because They Are)

Actively cultivate positive relationships. They are key to thriving and flourishing.

One of the greatest sources of happiness, joy, and well-being is positive relationships. Time spent with friends and loved ones yields a rich life beyond any benefits of material goods. In a study to identify the attributes of "Very Happy People"—the title of their 2002 article for the journal *Psychological Science*—Diener and Seligman found the most common trait of people whose survey results showed them to be consistently and significantly happier than their peers was a strong social network. The happiest among the 222 undergraduates participating in the research were "highly social," "more extroverted," and "more agreeable."[22] Their research results are certainly not isolated. Reporting on a 20-year analysis involving participants in the Framington Heart Study, British researchers found that people are happier when their close friends and family are happy, too, leading them to the view of "happiness, like health, as a collective phenomenon."[23] Another British researcher who surveyed 1,700 people on their level of life satisfaction and the quality and quantity of their friendships reported two key findings: Good friendships are worth investing time and effort to maintain, and the more friends you have the more likely you are to be happy. People who reported having five or fewer friends were more likely to be unhappy, whereas those with dozens of buddies reported much higher levels of life satisfaction.[24]

Summing up the research she and her colleagues conducted on the importance of social relationships, Lyubomirsky advises, "If you begin today to improve and cultivate your relationships, you will reap the gift of positive emotions. In turn, the enhanced feelings of happiness will help you attract more and higher-quality relationships, which will make you even happier, and so on, in a continuous positive feedback loop."[25]

Maintaining positive relationships requires time and effort on your part. Toward that end:

- Be the kind of spouse/partner, son/daughter, father/mother, and friend you would want to have—kind, supportive, positive, always willing to listen, and *always* ready to share a good laugh. We have shared plenty of laughs, even in the midst of hard work and deadlines. We take our work seriously, but not ourselves. We make a point of sharing small celebrations at dinner—for finishing a big chapter, delivering a presentation that met with a positive response from the audience, or hearing about the successes of a teacher who studied with the graduate program, for example. And during times of stress or difficulty, we remind each other to be kind to ourselves.
- Spread your happiness. Enjoy your time with the happy people in your life, and keep a ready smile and positive perspective on hand for the pessimists you know and love as well.
- Celebrate others' successes. Envy is counterproductive to positive relationships at best and emotionally crippling at its worst. When you set and pursue your own goals and benchmark your progress based on your own milestones, not those of others, you can more sincerely share in the joy when loved ones succeed.

- Make time for the ones you love. Even if you feel that your work and personal schedule is packed, it is essential to find "down time" to spend with friends and family. After years of living outside of England, Marcus made an effort to reconnect with friends from his teenage years: In our version of "getting the band back together again," we have agreed to team up to row in the Cambridge Town Bumps, a rowing competition in which boats race in single file with the aim of "bumping," or catching and passing, the teams in front of you. We all bring our families, relive our childhood adventures, and enjoy great company. We also have a big get-together at a favorite Cambridge restaurant. Now that we have reconnected, we stay in touch year-round via phone, e-mail, and Facebook.

8. Pursue Flow

Get lost in your enjoyment of a favorite pastime.

Mihalyi Csikszentmihalyi, the psychologist who collaborated with Martin Seligman at the dawn of positive psychology, came up with the term *flow* to describe the feeling of being completely immersed in a task and performing it well.[26] Flow is characterized by an energized focus and full involvement in the task and success in the endeavor. People experience flow when they harness positive emotions and all their attention and skills toward learning, progressing, and peak performance.

We will explore the experience of attaining flow more fully in the next chapter. For now, we want to underscore yet again the importance of directing your selective attention to activities you enjoy as a way to achieve greater happiness. Give yourself permission to focus exclusively on a favorite pastime or hobby and to get lost in your enjoyment of the task.

9. Pursue Smarter Goals

To experience the joy of accomplishment, set incremental goals to develop your skills and knowledge.

A powerful strategy for becoming positively smarter is to pursue smarter goals—short-term, measurable, achievable steps that set you on the path to achieve big, meaningful accomplishments. Identifying these smaller steps that pave the way to a larger goal allows you to develop your knowledge and skills and maintain a positive attitude as you make progress. Small celebrations along the way as you achieve those incremental milestones often provide the motivation to keep working until you achieve your major goal.

For example, Donna set a goal for becoming stronger at cycling so that we could go on a cycling holiday with friends: I started by riding a stationary bike at the gym with the short-term goal of increasing the length and difficulty of this workout every day. Before long, I was up to 30 minutes at fairly high resistance, and now I have set my sights on cycling for 45 minutes, gradually increasing the resistance to be ready to "head for the hills" on holiday. My workouts in the gym are translating into more pleasurable bike rides along the beach and paths as well. And the great thing about training on a stationary bike is that I could pass the time reading additional research for the book you are reading now!

Marcus has set a goal of running his second half marathon and a full marathon over the next year: So, while Donna is building her bike muscles, I have been steadily increasing my running strength and stamina. These goals have given great meaning and added satisfaction to our lives and improved our health. And we're having a great time along the way!

People of all ages can pursue—and achieve—smarter goals. Marcus's mother, Hazel Powell, had a vivid memory of a teacher in her childhood telling her she was not good at art. Throughout most of her life, she took that criticism to heart and avoided any artistic endeavor. Then at age 78, she attended a presentation by an artist at a local women's institute. At one point, the artist said, "Would anyone like to come up and help me and try your hand at a little bit of art?" With her heart pounding, Hazel went to the front of the room and picked up a paintbrush—and she's never looked back. She started taking art lessons at the high school, in the same classroom where Marcus once studied environmental science, and before long her paintings were on display in a local gallery. Her work has even been featured in international art magazines. The pursuit of her goal to build her skills and become an artist has given Hazel great pleasure every step of the way.

10. Enhance Your Resilience: Build Your Own Palmetto Fort

Let your prefrontal cortex steer your amygdala away from stress and anger.

In the early days of the Revolutionary War, patriots of the newly formed United States built a fort in Charleston, South Carolina, to withstand the onslaught of the British Navy. Its walls were built with palmetto logs, a wood so soft and pliable that it absorbed the blows from British cannons and stood strong until the battered ships were turned away from the harbor. We see the strength of the palmetto fort as an apt metaphor for how you can build your resilience and recover more quickly from emotional setbacks and losses.

In his research, Davidson identified connections between the prefrontal cortex, which is traditionally associated with executive functioning—that is, higher-order thinking—and the amygdala in the limbic system, which has long been considered the emotional center of the brain (see Figure 3.1). These connections are activated by emotional reactions of distress and anxiety. Davidson's experiments have demonstrated two crucial points:

1. People with greater activation on the left side of their prefrontal cortex recover more quickly from reacting to events that produce feelings of anger or fear. "Activity in the left prefrontal cortex actually shortens the period of amygdala activation, allowing the brain to bounce back from an upsetting experience."[27]
2. Through mindfulness training, or focusing their thoughts on calming down in an adverse situation, people can increase their

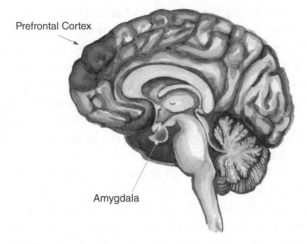

Prefrontal Cortex

Amygdala

Figure 3.1 Parts of the Brain That Support Resilience. © 2015 BrainSMART, Inc.

resilience "by weakening the chain of associations that keep us obsessing about and even wallowing in a setback."[28]

In other words, when confronted with a situation that makes you angry, upset, or stressed out, you can choose to hit the "pause" button rather than obsessing about those negative feelings and feeling worse and worse. Focus instead on how amazing it is that you have the power to control your emotions and steer them into more positive and productive territory. What's Important Now? Turning a bad situation into a WIN!

11. Untie the Knots That Bind: Free Yourself with Forgiveness

The best revenge is to invoke your power to rise above anger and resentment—to thrive!

Hanging on to anger, resentment, and hurt toward people who we think have hurt us can be quite an emotional burden and can pull us away from enjoying more positive experiences in life. Researchers have found that the process of forgiving can provide a powerful boost for our emotional and mental well-being. According to the customs of one tribe in Africa, whenever a baby is born in the village, all members of the community must resolve their resentments and arguments, each of which is represented by a knot in the fringe of their leather aprons. When they have settled their differences and untied all their knots, villagers can then attend the ceremony presenting the infant to the community.[29] This tradition shows a tremendous understanding of the importance of forgiving and letting go.

That's not to say that forgiveness is easy. It goes against our desire for justice and fairness to let go when we feel we have been wronged. Indeed, some transgressions, such as the physical and emotional toll of childhood abuse or neglect, may require a long road to recovery—but even in the direst circumstances, forgiveness provides a path "to transform anger [into] a summoning of peace," in the words of Judith Orloff, author of *Emotional Freedom*. And for lesser slights, letting go of anger and resentment offers the best revenge, Orloff suggests—"your success, happiness, and the triumph of not giving vindictive people any dominion over your peace of mind."[30]

As with increasing your resilience, putting emotional injuries behind you requires thinking about your feelings. Acknowledge and address your feelings of anger and hurt. It may help to talk through those feelings with your partner, a friend, or a therapist. Or you may want to write about them in a journal or a letter to yourself or to the person behind the transgression. Then, consciously take charge of shifting your emotions in a more positive direction. Recognize your strengths to move beyond painful feelings and to focus on what is good about yourself and your life.

12. Move Your Body, Boost Your Mood

Physical activity provides a reliable antidote to stress and anxiety.

Regular physical activity has been shown to alleviate depression, reduce stress, and diminish feelings of anxiety. The mood-enhancing effects of exercise are typically felt during or within minutes of completing a workout.[31] Scientists continue to explore why physical activity elevates emotional well-being—maybe because it increases serotonin levels or provides an uplifting sense of accomplishment—but whatever the mechanism(s), exercise provides a ready and reliable mood boost. In Chapter 7, we will examine in greater detail the current research about the benefits of exercise. For now, let's focus on its ability to replace stress and negativity with feelings of calm contentment. Have you just finished a difficult phone conversation with a client? Have you been staring at the computer screen for so long the text is starting to blur? Is the noise from the construction zone next door grating at your nerves? Take an exercise break and you will return feeling energized, focused, and in a much more positive mindset!

13. Smile, and Your Brain Smiles with You

When life is jolly rotten, there's something you've forgotten, and that's to laugh and smile and dance and sing.—Monty Python

Marcus recalls this encounter while doing a presentation in the Deep South: I was fully involved in conveying the material, enjoying myself but apparently coming across as a serious, unsmiling Englishman. A voice from the back of the room boomed out, "Boy, are you happy?" I paused and said, "Yes." "Well, then," responded the disembodied voice, "tell your darn face." I joined the audience in a round of laughter and from then on felt free to relax and smile.

Smiling may be both a cause and effect of positive emotions. The brain receives neurochemical cues from the nerves and muscles in your face about how you're feeling. In *Emotional Intelligence 2.0*, Bradberry and Greaves note that "when you laugh and smile, your face sends signals to your brain that you are happy."[32] If you smile, you can often boost your mood.

14. Play to Your Peak Strengths

Recognizing your special talents can be rejuvenating.

Becoming positively smarter is about learning new knowledge and developing new skills, but it also involves parlaying your strengths to maximum impact. People are often at their happiest when they are immersed in activities they enjoy and are good at. You might find great pleasure in baking your special muffins that always get rave reviews from family and friends or in framing the beautiful photographs you took while traveling. Whenever Donna travels to a university town, she tries to arrange her schedule so she can spend some time immersed in research and reading at the education library: That is my way of indulging in my love of learning and sharing what I discover—and there's always something new—with others.

We use this concept of playing to our strengths when working together. In teamwork it is important to value differences and notice how marvelously team members' talents complement each other's and compensate for weaknesses. When we are writing together, Donna's strengths are in pulling together research, stories, and examples from her work in education and psychology. Marcus's peak strengths are gathering current data from many fields of science and business and creating practical strategies based on that research. Both of us recognize that we are not so good at bureaucratic tasks that involve a lot of procedures.

In the graduate studies program we codeveloped, many teachers have enjoyed learning about themselves and their signature strengths. Some teachers have even reported feeling transformed and rejuvenated by identifying their strengths and talents, and they say they have translated this exercise successfully for use with their students.

What are your signature strengths? In what activities do you find satisfaction in performing well? Would you enjoy further developing these skills and polishing your strengths and talents?

15. Practice the Art of Treasuring

Every second is a diamond if you choose to let it shine.

At any given moment, even in the most hectic of days, you can choose to slow down and treasure what you are experiencing. Start your morning out right by hugging a loved one, or sipping your coffee on the patio and enjoying your surroundings. Take a break from a busy workday to go for a stroll or run. Turn just another evening into a special occasion by inviting friends over to try out a new recipe. Break out the photo albums and recall fond memories of past adventures. Call a distant friend or relative out of the blue and enjoy a good laugh together. Every second can be a diamond if you choose to let it shine.

When we were first married, we moved into a smallish condo with no yard to speak of. One night we were dining outside on our tiny patio, when we were visited by a pair of cardinals. The male was so resplendent in red and the pair of them were so stately that we felt as if we had been visited by royalty. The birds became such regular visitors that we started calling them Mr. and Mrs. Wolsey. We took delight in their presence and commenting, only partly in jest, about how their interactions provided a fine role model for couples' communication. We followed the progress of their family life, how they patiently gathered materials and assembled their nest, and how they would come to rest on a nearby tree as if to reflect on a good day's work. We would see them out with their youngsters and imagined that they must be teaching them how to find food and avoid predators. The birds would execute backflips and swoops off the edge of the roof, and after a couple of demonstrations, the younger redbirds would follow suit. We truly treasured those idle evenings observing the Wolseys and the feelings of contentment that came from just being in those moments.

How to Be Less Happy More of the Time

Daydream—a lot. Buy the expensive car instead of investing in memorably great experiences with loved ones. Procrastinate about being kind. Focus on acquiring things. Spend as little time as possible with friends and family. Take for granted all that you have to be grateful for. Take joy in the misfortunes of others. Be a perfectionist. Criticize. Hold grudges. Whine, blame, complain. Allow yourself to be consumed by your problems. Steer clear of aerobic exercise and strength training. Don't read, learn, and expand your mind.

Maintain Your Positive Focus by Playing Your ACE

The Focused Fifteen presented in this chapter offer a wide variety of everyday strategies for becoming positively smarter. To maintain an optimistic outlook that you will be able to achieve your goals, play your ACE as a sure bet to rely on three areas involving practical metacognition that are mostly under your control:

- **Appreciate** the caring people and positive experiences in your life. The happiest people we know are extremely skilled at appreciating the people around them and the experiences they have day by day. This focus on appreciation amplifies positivity and produces even more positive interactions, relationships, and experiences.
- **Complete** 80/20 tasks, the 20 percent of activities that produce 80 percent of positive results. By focusing on the most effective strategies for becoming positively smarter, you will greatly increase your chances of attaining your goals. Which of the topics presented in this book do you need to work on improving the most? Which of these strategies have proven to be most effective for you? Those are your 80/20 tasks.
- **Enhance** your knowledge and skills. In the next section, we will explore how neuroplasticity enables us to keep learning new ideas throughout our lives. By focusing on improving your skills, knowledge, and positive attitude, you will become increasingly more effective and more productive, which in turn feeds into your level of happiness.

By bringing these three overarching ideas together, you can target your thoughts, energies, and actions in an extremely productive way. Marcus has constructed a daily planner to underscore his appreciation for completing important tasks and enhancing key skills. It is rewarding at the end of each day to see progress in those areas. By deliberately planning for and achieving progress in these three areas, you too can increase your opportunities for becoming positively smarter.

Notes

1   The Huffington Post. "Professor Richard J. Davidson: 'Happiness Is a Skill That Can Be Learned.'" HuffPost Healthy Living, January 23, 2014. Retrieved from http://www.huffingtonpost.com/2014/01/23/richard-j-davidson-davos_n_4636683.html

2   Matthew A. Killingsworth and Daniel T. Gilbert. "A Wandering Mind Is an Unhappy Mind." *Science*, November 12, 2010, p. 932.

3   Ibid.

4   Martin E. P. Seligman. 2011. *Flourish: A Visionary New Understanding of Happiness and Well-Being.* New York: Free Press, p. 33.

5   Richard J. Davidson, with Sharon Begley. 2012. *The Emotional Life of Your Brain.* New York: Hudson Street Press, p. 89.

6   Robert J. Sternberg, Linda Jarvin, and Elena L. Grigorenko. 2009. *Teaching for Wisdom, Intelligence, Creativity, and Success.* Thousand Oaks, CA: Corwin Press; Howard Gardner. 2006. *Multiple Intelligences: New Horizons in Theory and Practice* (rev. ed.). New York: Basic Books.

7   Travis Bradberry and Jean Greaves. 2009. *Emotional Intelligence 2.0.* San Diego, CA: TalentSmart, pp. 20–21.

8   Bradberry and Greaves, pp. 7–8.

9   Barbara Fredrickson. 2009. *Positivity: Top-Notch Research Reveals the 3-1 Ratio That Will Change Your Life.* New York: Three Rivers Press, p. 9.

10 Alexandra B. Morrison, Merissa Goolsarran, Scott L. Rogers, and Amishi P. Jha. "Taming a Wandering Attention: Short-Form Mindfulness Training in Student Cohorts." *Frontiers in Human Neuroscience*, January 2014, Article 897.

11 Mihalyi Csikszentmihalyi. 1997. *Finding Flow: The Psychology of Engagement with Everyday Life.* New York: Basic Books, pp. 27–28.

12 Jon Hamilton. "Think You're Multitasking? Think Again." NPR, October 2, 2008. Retrieved from http://www.npr.org/templates/story/story.php?storyId=95256794

13 Scott Barry Kaufman. "Mind Wandering: A New Personal Intelligence Perspective." *Scientific American* Blogs: Beautiful Minds, September 25, 2013. Retrieved from http://blogs.scientificamerican.com/beautiful-minds/2013/09/25/mind-wandering-a-new-personal-intelligence-perspective/

14 Martin Seligman. 2002. *Authentic Happiness: Using the New Positive Psychology to Realize Your Potential for Lasting Fulfillment.* New York: Simon & Schuster.

15 David Hecht. "The Neural Basis of Optimism and Pessimism." *Experimental Neurobiology*, 22(3), September 2013, 173–199. doi: 10.5607/en.2013.22.3.173

16 Viktor Frankl. 1946/1984. *Man's Search for Meaning* (Ilse Lasch, trans.). New York: Washington Square Press, pp. 94–95.

17 K. E. Buchanan and A. Bardi. "Acts of Kindness and Acts of Novelty Affect Life Satisfaction." *Journal of Social Psychology*, *150*(3), 2010, 235–237; Sonja Lyubomirsky. 2007. *The How of Happiness: A New Approach to Getting the Life You Want*. New York: Penguin; Northern Arizona University Research. "Two Effective Strategies for Increasing Happiness." Retrieved from http://nau.edu/Research/Feature-Stories/Two-Effective-Strategies-for-Increasing-Happiness/; K. Otake, S. Shimai, J. Tanaka-Matsumi, and colleagues. "Happy People Become Happier Through Kindness: A Counting Kindnesses Intervention." *Journal of Happiness Studies*, September 2006, 361–375. Retrieved from http://www.ncbi.nlm.nih.gov/pmc/articles/PMC1820947/

18 Alex Dixon. "Kindness Makes You Happy ... And Happiness Makes You Kind." Greater Good: The Science of a Meaningful Life (University of California, Berkeley), September 6, 2011. Retrieved from http://greatergood.berkeley.edu/article/item/kindness_makes_you_happy_and_happiness_makes_you_kind

19 M. J. Poulin, S. L. Brown, A. J. Dillard, and D. M. Smith. "Giving to Others and the Association Between Stress and Mortality." *American Journal of Public Health*, *103*(9), September 2013, 1649–1655.

20 Seligman, *Flourish*, p. 21.

21 William C. Compton and Edward Hoffman. 2013. *Positive Psychology: The Science of Happiness and Flourishing* (2nd ed.). Belmont, CA: Wadsworth, p. 236.

22 Ed Diener and Martin E. P. Seligman. "Very Happy People." *Psychological Science*, *13*(1), January 2002, 81–84. doi: 10.1111/1467-9280.00415

23 James H. Fowler and Nicholas A. Christakis. "Dynamic Spread of Happiness in a Large Social Network: Longitudinal Analysis over 20 Years in the Framington Heart Study." *The BMJ*, December 5, 2008. Retrieved from http://www.bmj.com/content/337/bmj.a2338

24 Fiona Macrae. "The Secret to Happiness? Having at Least 10 Good Friends." *The Daily Mail Online*, October 23, 2008. Retrieved from http://www.dailymail.co.uk/news/article-1079997/The-secret-happiness-Having-10-good-friends.html

25 Lyubomirsky, pp. 138–139.

26 Mihalyi Csikszentmihalyi. 1997. *Finding Flow: The Psychology of Engagement with Everyday Life*. New York: Basic Books.

27 Richard J. Davidson. "Tired of Feeling Bad? The New Science of Feelings Can Help." *Newsweek*, February 21, 2012. Retrieved from http://www.newsweek.com/tired-feeling-bad-new-science-feelings-can-help-65743

28 Ibid.

29   Carla Hannaford. 2007. *Smart Moves: Why Learning Is Not All in Your Head* (2nd ed.). Salt Lake City, UT: Great River Books, p. 228.

30   Judith Orloff. "The Power of Forgiveness: Why Revenge Doesn't Work." *Psychology Today*, September 8, 2011. Retrieved from http://www.psychologytoday.com/blog/emotional-freedom/201109/the-power-forgiveness-even-911

31   Kirsten Weir. "The Exercise Effect." *American Psychological Association Monitor*, *42*(11), December 2011. Retrieved from http://www.apa.org/monitor/2011/12/exercise.aspx

32   Bradberry and Greaves, p. 114.

4

Working Toward Achieving
Your Goals

"Thinking about intelligence as changeable and malleable, rather than stable and fixed, results in greater academic achievement, especially for people whose groups bear the burden of negative stereotypes about their intelligence."

—American Psychological Association[1]

There are many ways of becoming positively smarter—outlooks, abilities, and strategies you can develop to increase your happiness, achievement, and physical well-being. Psychologist Robert Sternberg is a leading proponent of widening the scope of education to teach students the most useful skills and attitudes they can wield to achieve meaningful success in their lives—not just analytical intelligence, but creativity, a commonsense approach to problem solving, and the wisdom to act ethically and in a way that balances the interests of all involved. All of these attributes are "modifiable and dynamic," Sternberg underscores. "One is not born with a fixed level of wisdom, intelligence, or creativity, but rather develops these attributes over time."[2] He shares a personal story about the impact in education of focusing on one of these abilities to the exclusion of others:

Positively Smarter: Science and Strategies for Increasing Happiness, Achievement, and Well-Being, First Edition. Marcus Conyers and Donna Wilson.
© 2015 John Wiley & Sons, Inc. Published 2015 by John Wiley & Sons, Inc.

As a freshman at Yale, I was extremely eager to major in psychology because I had done so poorly on IQ tests as a child and wanted to understand why. I took the introductory psychology course and got a C. My professor at one point stared at me and commented that there was a famous Sternberg in the field of psychology (Saul Sternberg) and that it was obvious there would not be another one.[3]

The "other" Sternberg looked back on that college experience more than three decades later when he returned to Yale as a chaired professor and president of the American Psychological Association, noting the differences between the skills needed to ace an introductory college course and those needed to succeed in his chosen field. His story illustrates the difference that dedication, persistence, and hard work can make in achieving one's potential, and his life's work has provided a framework for an effective teaching approach to equip students with a range of skills to help them succeed in school and in life.

Realizing Our Potential

When we say that virtually everyone has the potential to become positively smarter, we mean that they have the capacity to make steady progress over time. There is no certainty of success. Not all children who come to school with the capacity to become readers achieve that outcome, as many do not experience the support at home or the high-quality instruction at school they need to develop those skills. Not every person who starts jogging becomes a marathoner. Not every invention makes its inventor a millionaire. Potential does not automatically translate into expert performance, nor does it guarantee a positive outcome. But we can say this with certainty: You will not achieve your goals if you aren't motivated to do the work necessary to attain them.

Neurocognitive plasticity gives nearly every child the potential to learn how to read. Their parents and teachers help children learn the necessary reading skills, convey the attitude and outlook that they can learn to read, and foster motivation that reading is both essential and enjoyable. Adults also help children become readers by giving them ample exposure to language and opportunities to hone their reading skills. Children do the work of learning and practicing reading skills to become increasingly fluent readers with ever-expanding vocabularies.

Along the same lines, a person who starts jogging only becomes a marathoner if she is sufficiently committed and motivated to undergo the rigorous, ongoing training necessary to get in shape for long-distance running and maintain that form.

In the case of an inventor, it takes hard work and dedication to translate an idea into reality, and even then there are no guarantees the invention will find a wide market. Likewise, a novelist can finish a book, a composer a symphony, and a sculptor a statue without ultimately achieving widespread recognition for the true worth of their creations. Our focus in this text is on how you can achieve your potential by setting goals and working to achieve them—to aim for your individual best. Table 4.1 offers an action assessment so you can consider how well you currently use effective strategies for working toward your goals.

Table 4.1 Action Assessment: Working Toward Your Goals

On a daily basis, how often do you …	*Almost never*	*Sometimes*	*Frequently*	*Consistently*
1. Move outside your comfort zone to take positive risks.				
2. Set your sights on mastering new skills and knowledge rather than relying on external performance measures.				
3. Identify and build on your strengths.				

(continued)

94

Table 4.1 Action Assessment: Working Toward Your Goals (*cont'd*)

On a daily basis, how often do you ...	Almost never	Sometimes	Frequently	Consistently
4. Establish step-by-step objectives to work toward achieving larger goals.				
5. Pace yourself to head off burnout.				
6. Aim for progress, not perfection.				
7. Picture your success to maintain focus, motivation, and momentum.				
8. Employ effective strategies to improve retention of important information.				

"Natural" Talent vs. Deliberate Practice

We touched on a common myth about achievement in the introduction—that high performance is largely the product of innate talent. Different versions of this assumption pop up all over the place. Mozart was a child prodigy. This or that athlete is a "natural." An intellectual couple are "geniuses"; therefore, their child must be a "genius," too. These labels get thrown around a lot under the guise that some people are genetically destined for greatness.

This myth does a disservice to both those people who have excelled in their chosen endeavors and the rest of us who set high goals for ourselves. In the first case, the assumption that some people are successful just because they are innately gifted neglects giving them credit for their hard work and many hours of intense practice. Let's hear a big round of applause for the hardest working people at the top of their fields. They earned it! And, in the bargain, let's put aside the implicit message to the rest of us: Don't bother. You don't have what it takes. The reality is, you do—but recognize that it's not always going to be an easy ride.

In other words, we need to put aside the misperception that the highest performers rely solely on talent. As Geoffrey Colvin notes in an article in *Fortune* magazine, decades of research can be summarized in a simple conclusion: "Nobody is great without work."[4] Psychology professor K. Anders Ericsson has put forth the proposition that outstanding performance is the product of hard work and lots of it—in the range of 5,000 to 10,000 hours of practice to become an "expert" in any endeavor. In an article in the *Harvard Business Review*, Ericsson and his colleagues cite research that finds little evidence of natural talent and no significant link between IQ and excellence in fields ranging from chess and sports competition to medicine. In short, they argue, "experts are always made, not born." They explain:

> The development of genuine expertise requires struggle, sacrifice, and honest, often painful self-assessment. There are no shortcuts. It will take you at least a decade to achieve expertise, and you will need to invest that time wisely, by engaging in "deliberate" practice— practice that focuses on tasks beyond your current level of competence and comfort.[5]

Ericsson and his colleagues define deliberate practice as hard work that "entails considerable, specific, and sustained efforts to do something you can't do well—or even at all."[6] This work involves both hands-on practice and thinking about how to improve your skills, on your own and with the guidance of an experienced teacher, mentor, or coach. Deliberate practice dedicated to developing your knowledge, skills, and abilities need not take over your life—the most celebrated athletes and artists typically practice two to four hours a day, usually in the morning when they are rested and ready to tackle tough mental challenges—but it must be focused and rigorous and aim for continuous improvement. Committing yourself to deliberate practice "puts brains in your muscles," the authors suggest.[7]

In earlier research, Ericsson, Krampe, and Tesch-Romer differentiated deliberate practice from work, in which people are paid for performance and tend to rely on entrenched methods, and play, in which people engage with no explicit goal just because they enjoy it. They define deliberate practice as "activities that have been specially designed to improve the current level of performance."[8] There are no immediate rewards for engaging in deliberate practice, and it is not inherently enjoyable. In fact, people engaging in this form of intensive training must be extremely motivated to persist through seemingly endless repetitions of specific tasks designed to overcome weaknesses. Deliberate practice is highly individual and geared to specific needs, and it provides opportunities to explore alternative, unproven methods of gaining expertise. People who set out to become experts in their fields must overcome time, resource, and effort constraints; they must be willing and able to devote a great deal of time and money to their pursuits and to build extraordinary stamina. Over time, this expertise accumulates in long-term memory, as demonstrated by chess masters' ability to predict and respond to an opponent's future moves or a pianist's ability to perform a complex piece seemingly without effort. Thus, what seems to be innate talent is in fact the product of hard work and practice to steadily improve knowledge and abilities.

Many other researchers and authors who have studied what sets successful people apart have come to similar conclusions about the rewards of extraordinary effort and persistence. In short, doing the hard work to develop a talent that seems to come naturally takes years and requires unflagging devotion, motivation, and sacrifice. Mozart gained a reputation as a child prodigy because he began to pursue his love of music at an early age and had intensive training. Ericsson and colleagues share the perspective of golfing great Sam Snead, who was dubbed "the best natural player ever." Snead shrugged off that label: "People always said I had a natural swing. They thought I wasn't a hard worker. But when I was young, I'd play and practice all day, then practice more at night by my car's headlights. My hands bled. Nobody worked harder at golf than I did."[9]

Motivation to Take Positive Risks

Beyond a willingness to do the hard work and learning to develop your skills, knowledge, and physical abilities, achieving more of your potential requires a willingness to take risks—to try something new, to believe in your ability to succeed, and to make a difference for yourself and others. "Few do what they know they should, what they know they could, what they know truly matters," writes Bill Jensen in his essay on "The Biggest Distance in the World."[10]

A crucial ingredient in this new "recipe for success" is the need to keep pushing yourself to take on new challenges, to move outside your comfort zone to try things you're not sure you can accomplish. To achieve one's potential sometimes means NOT playing it safe—by trying something or sticking with something even if it's not a sure bet. In *The Winner's Brain*, Brown and Fenske note that successful people "try to better their situation (and sometimes the world) by taking risks that are substantial enough that they have a personal stake in the outcome, yet more gratifying than if they sat on the sidelines playing it safe." In short, successful people "know when to dive in headfirst and when to walk away."[11] To be able to continually challenge yourself requires developing self-awareness about your talents, strengths, and learning preferences.

Any goal that entails hard work and a long-term commitment to attain it also requires motivation to stick with it. There are all sorts of incentives and motivators for high performance, many of them external—getting good grades in school, earning a promotion or pay raise on the job, or losing weight because you want to look good at your child's wedding. The only problem with these types of external rewards is that they have a limited impact unless they are aligned with your internal motivation, also known as intrinsic or self-motivation.

Psychologists refer to goals that are driven by external motivations as *performance goals* in contrast to *mastery goals*, which refer to desires to develop and improve skills and abilities.[12] Is your primary motivation in taking a Spanish class to get an A or to learn the language well enough to communicate when you travel? In her book *Succeed: How We Can Reach Our Goals*, social psychologist Heidi Grant Halvorson distinguishes between "be good" (performance) and "get better" (mastery) goals.[13] She suggests that performance goals can be quite motivating and notes that the highest performers in school and in the workplace are often driven by the desire to be the best. But these goals are intertwined with feelings of self-worth: When people are driven by the desire to be the best in comparison to others, they feel good about themselves when they succeed and bad when they don't—and are more likely to give up rather than persist through difficult challenges. That's why performance goals may ultimately "lead to the lowest achievement, along with a heavy dose of disappointment and self-doubt," Grant Halvorson cautions.[14] In comparison, people pursuing mastery goals are more likely to keep trying and be less daunted by setbacks, more likely to ask for help and try different strategies if at first they don't succeed, and more likely to find pleasure in making progress and thus continue working through the steps to achieve a complex task or long-term goal.

Motivation is a topic of fascination for psychologists who have devised all sorts of experiments through the years to study what makes us tick, what moves us to action. These experiments have consistently found that intrinsic motivation is much more powerful than external rewards. As Brown and Fenske note, "it seems that productivity and external rewards are inversely proportional after a certain threshold." They summarize the research on motivation:

To begin with, extrinsic rewards tend to encourage people to focus narrowly on a task, to do it as quickly as possible, and to take few risks. They focus on getting the prize and less on the creative process of reaching the goal. Second, they often begin to feel as if they are being controlled by the reward, so they tend to be less invested and less performance-oriented than if they were doing it for the sense of accomplishment or even a compliment from the boss. The less self-determined they feel, the more their creative juices dry up. And lastly, focus on extrinsic rewards can erode intrinsic interest. People who see themselves as working for money, approval, or competitive success find their tasks less pleasurable, and therefore have more trouble getting them done.[15]

Working for external rewards can only get you so far if the object of those rewards is out of sync with your intrinsic motivations. Thus, when teachers encourage students to look inside themselves for motivation to learn instead of looking for outside rewards, they are guiding students to develop a mindset that will serve them well throughout their years in school and beyond as adults. For many high-performing employees, the sense of satisfaction over a job well done often outweighs financial bonuses and recognition from their bosses. Teachers, as just one example, know this well firsthand!

Many Americans are discovering the joys and motivations to succeed by striking out on their own in the working world, pursuing an entrepreneurial path by becoming consultants, independent contractors, and small business owners. Being your own boss requires a commitment to hard work and the motivation to develop the abilities you will need to succeed—not just the skills of your trade or profession, but an understanding of financial management, human resources, marketing, and customer service. To help maintain our home, we rely on the services of a handyman named John. He's helped us with projects from installing new shelves to fixing balky appliances. We are amazed at his abilities and range of knowledge about home repairs. John says he does spend a lot of time learning new skills and maintaining his knowledge of building code requirements. However, he told us that his biggest challenge in starting his own handyman business was developing his "people skills" and getting the hang of developing cost estimates for his customers. Lately, he said, he's most proud not of his carpentry or painting skills, but of his newly developed ability to use basic bookkeeping software! His motivation to run his own business fuels his persistence to continually develop new skills.

Finding "Flow"

Accomplishing your potential often entails hard work and determination to develop skills and abilities to that transcendent level that you lose yourself in the pleasure of accomplishment. A competitive runner is so transfixed by achieving the perfect rhythm that she crosses the finish line before she knows it. A potter in his studio looks up to realize a whole day has passed while he has been captivated by his work. A gardener shakes the dirt from her gloves as she arises after hours of planting and landscaping to admire, somewhat in surprise, all that she has achieved in one afternoon. Mihalyi Csikszentmihalyi came up with the term *flow* to describe the feeling of being completely immersed in a task and performing it well. Flow is characterized by an energized focus and full involvement in the task and success in the endeavor. People experience flow when they harness positive emotions and all their attention and skills toward learning, progressing, and peak performance. Athletes refer to being "in the zone" or "in the groove." In education, a whole class may experience flow when the teacher and students are so caught up with a learning activity that they groan in disappointment to hear the bell ring at the end of class.

Achieving the state of flow requires a balance between level of ability and interest (you're pursuing something you find engaging and motivating and you're good at it) and challenge (the task at hand is not so easy that you lose interest and not so tough that you grow frustrated). Csikszentmihalyi notes that enjoyment is a crucial aspect of flow:

> Usually the more difficult a mental task, the harder it is to concentrate on it. But when a person likes what he does and is motivated to do it, focusing the mind becomes effortless even when the objective difficulties are great.[16]

A positive outlook and environment are also essential:

> When a person is anxious or worried, for example, the step to flow often seems too far, and one retreats to a less challenging situation

instead of trying to cope. .... The flow experience acts as a magnet for learning—that is, for developing new levels of challenges and skills.[17]

The concept of flow conveys the intrinsic reward that comes from setting your sights high and then committing to the effort needed to reach that level. Achieving one's life goals is hard work that often entails overcoming setbacks to keep progressing. You are more likely to stay on course if you are engaged and motivated along the way and if you enjoy and find fulfillment in what you are doing. Csikszentmihalyi uses the term *autotelic personality* to describe a person "who generally does things for their own sake, rather than in order to achieve some later external goal."[18] High performers may be described as autotelic in that area where they excel, but what motivates them may vary widely. Mathematicians and scientists are motivated by curiosity and their excitement to explore and solve puzzles. Engineers, musicians, and artists are moved by the desire to create. Teachers, nurses, doctors, and social workers attain internal satisfaction by helping others. Successful athletes may be most motivated by the spirit of competition—the desire to win. What moves you? By identifying your source of internal motivation, you can more effectively identify the pursuits that you are willing to work hard to attain.

Putting Your Will to Work

Becoming positively smarter is an ambitious pursuit that may provide many benefits in your personal and professional life, but nobody said it would be easy. Making the most of your neuroplasticity to improve your outlook, knowledge, skills, and well-being is hard work and will require persistent effort and strong, internal motivation. Roy Baumeister's research on willpower offers some insights on developing the discipline and dedication you will need to accomplish your goals. A key finding is that your supply of willpower is finite: You only have so much to expend across all the tasks and challenges you undertake. If you exert a lot of self-control in one area of your life, you have less to expend in other areas. For example, if your work requires extreme discipline and focus, you may feel more inclined to kick back and relax in your personal life. Or as Baumeister and Tierney write in *Willpower: Rediscovering the Greatest Human Strength*, "You use the same supply of willpower to deal with frustrating traffic, tempting food, annoying colleagues, demanding bosses, pouting children. Resisting dessert at lunch leaves you with less willpower to praise your boss's awful haircut."[19]

The good news is that you can "power up" your willpower. In experiments on improving physical fitness, study habits, and personal money management, participants increased their stamina to resist temptation and stay focused in other areas as well.[20] Consciously focusing your attention and energy to accomplish important tasks can pay dividends in strengthening your resolve to take on other challenges.

You needn't rely solely on willpower to accomplish your goals. Establishing a strong support system and employing some effective strategies for working smarter can lighten the load. Adopting these outlooks and tactics can help bolster your will to persist in the work needed to develop new knowledge, implement new skill sets, and strengthen your abilities.

Identify and build on your strengths Hallowell recommends that people consider what they do best in deciding what endeavors to pursue: "You ought to do most what you do best. It's amazing how many people spend years trying to get good at what they're bad at instead of getting better at what they're good at."[21] Or as Brown and Fenske put it: "You might have the potential of becoming a great public speaker, an amazing parent, or an incredible teacher, but if you don't recognize those abilities within yourself, you won't take the time to develop those natural talents."[22]

Establish smart goals You may have an audacious goal—to learn to play the piano, to launch a successful business, or to eliminate the happy clutter in the home where you raised your family so you can move across the country to pursue new challenges in retirement.

Accomplishing a big goal becomes much more doable if you set smaller, measurable goals that you can monitor and adjust as necessary to move steadily in the right direction. For example, you will practice the piano at least an hour four times a week in order to learn two new pieces every month while improving on your existing repertoire. You will research the market for your business idea, develop a formal business plan, and meet with a mentor to review your ideas by the end of the summer. You will sort your belongings into "garage sale," "donations," "recycling," and "keep" piles closet by closet and room by room over the next two months—and then go through the "keep" pile one last time. Short-term goals help you make steady progress and achieve incremental aims to build confidence, stay positive, and bolster motivation (and celebrate along the way to maintain your motivation!), while long-term goals help you stay focused on the ultimate prize.[23]

Pace yourself Along the same lines, it will be helpful to set timelines for accomplishing your goals that recognize the limits of your attention, time, and stamina. If you're conducting a research project, for example, you'll probably get more accomplished if you spend two hours at the library, take a break for lunch and a brisk walk in the fresh air, and then return for two more hours at the library than if you spend six hours on library research without a break. In teaching, we refer to "chunking" lessons, or planning learning activities in segments that correspond to students' optimal attention spans, based on their age. Young children learn most effectively when presented with smaller chunks of information interspersed with hands-on learning activities to reinforce the learning. Adult attention spans may be longer, but not infinite. A recent study found that employees experience more flow during the workday if they take time away from work to "refresh" with fun and relaxing activities.[24] It seems that all work and no play really can make us duller. As we will note in Chapter 7, a slightly different dynamic applies to building your physical skills: You need to build your stamina and endurance by ratcheting up the intensity of your workouts over time. To avoid burning out and abandoning your goals, move forward at an ambitious, but measured, pace.

Aim for progress, not perfection In Donna's presentations to doctoral students at the Global Conference hosted each summer by Nova Southeastern University, a message that resonates is to "create first and edit later." Think about this example: You've got a big report to write. You wake up excited about the good news you'll be sharing, and you think of key points to share all the way to work, but when you sit down in front of the computer, all those great ideas vanish. If only you could come up with a brilliant first sentence, you think, the rest will flow easily. Our prescription: Forget about your intro for now and just jot down your main ideas. Once you have *something* in writing, it will be much easier to shape it, expand it, revise it, and come up with the best possible intro.

Picture your success This is another popular maxim with the doctoral students I coach: Think about the ways you will be able to make a difference in the world when you complete your studies. Setting your sights on a positive future is an effective motivator. Embrace your capacity for change. As we noted in Chapter 3, a positive outlook can mean the difference between persisting when the going gets tough and giving up.

CIA in Action: Productivity in the Workplace

In Chapter 2, we introduced the CIA (control–influence–acknowledge) model to help you stay focused on achieving your goals. Let's consider how you can apply this model on the job to maintain motivation and enhance personal productivity.

Control: Focus on completing important tasks and implementing strategies to increase achievement and productivity.

Influence: Your beliefs about your abilities, achievement, and performance and your contribution to the achievement and performance of others (as a team member, assistant, or supervisor).

Acknowledge: Challenges that are beyond your control. For example, you may be required to complete tasks that might be considered less productive, such as reports that do not contribute directly to achievement and interactions with colleagues who are unproductive, uncommitted, and/or pessimistic. Minimize your time and energy spent in these areas to the extent possible to maintain your motivation and focus on progress.

Getting Gritty as a Path to Achievement

Taken together, these strategies can help enhance grit, a key attribute of people who succeed in achieving ambitious goals through hard work and determination. Angela Duckworth and her colleagues define *grit* simply as "perseverance and passion for long-term goals."[25] These researchers developed a questionnaire to assess this trait in subjects pursuing achievement in three settings: students pursuing degrees at Ivy League schools, West Point cadets, and contestants in the National Spelling Bee. The subjects who earned the best grades, made it through the tough first year of the military academy, and advanced through multiple rounds of the spelling bee were assessed as having high levels of grit. These findings lead to the conclusion that success is not just about developing talent but "the sustained and focused application of talent over time."[26]

As with other attributes that we've explored thus far, it is possible to improve your grit and, as a result, to become more persistent and determined in working toward achieving your goals. Grant Halvorson notes that:

People who lack grit, more often than not, believe that they just don't have the innate abilities successful people have. If that describes your own thinking ... well, there's no way to put this nicely: you are wrong. ... Effort, planning, persistence, and developing good strategies are what it really takes to succeed. Embracing this knowledge will not only help you see yourself and your goals more accurately, but also do wonders for your grit.[27]

Psychologist Sian Beilock has studied the research on how athletes, business people, and students can set aside these kinds of self-doubts to achieve peak performance in their various arenas. The most effective remedies to avoid "choking" in high-pressure situations include intensive practice so that key skills become second nature and acknowledgment of and preparation for performance pressures, such as the stress of competing before a crowd or of doing well on a high-stakes test.[28] Among the obstacles that stand in the way of choke-free performance are the biases and false beliefs of others—that women can't do math, for example, or that children from disadvantaged backgrounds can't excel in school. It is possible to confront and replace those biases with the confidence that comes with achievement through persistent effort.

Donna often feels these pressures when she is preparing to speak at an educational conference: Anticipating my presentation prior to going on stage and in the first few minutes, I often feel a bit anxious. One strategy I've found helpful is to practice the presentation several times with specific focus on memorizing the first minute of my speech. I have learned to consciously focus on my higher purpose for doing this work—to add to the greater good by supporting educators and communities with current knowledge and a practical approach to flourishing in school and in life. It helps to revisit the positive risks I have taken in my work and to recall the impact I have seen in applying the approach I am about to introduce to my audience.

Practice Makes Progress for Young Readers

An early example of proceeding with the power of positive determination can be seen in young children learning to read. As we noted previously, the reading readiness of children entering schools spans a wide range, based largely on their early exposure to language and literacy. Children who seem to have a natural affinity for reading have likely been immersed in language at home since early infancy—being spoken to and encouraged to speak and being read to daily. The good news is that children who arrive in kindergarten unprepared to "do school" can catch up with their peers. In fact, education professor Richard Allington makes the case that 90 percent or more of all students have the academic potential to read on grade level, although many fail to do so.[29] To fulfill their potential to become fluent readers, these students need the opportunity afforded by intensive, high-quality reading instruction. In short, they need lots and lots of practice reading. One proven strategy for improving reading skills is encouraging children to read materials at their independent reading level—that is, texts that they can read with 95 to 98 percent accuracy. They can read at this level without struggling and becoming frustrated so that they continue to develop fluency and improve their reading skills. In effect, these children can experience flow in reading and begin to discover that reading can be a pleasurable activity.

Build Your "Memory Muscle" to Make the Most of Your Work

An advantage that "experts" have in their chosen fields is that their extensive practice and work in their endeavors have woven a great deal of knowledge into their memories. For example, Beilock notes that chess masters' "enormous amount of practice ... allows them to see meaningful patterns in the board that less skilled players can see. These patterns can help masters think ahead ten moves whereas a less skilled player can only think three moves out."[30]

Thus, what seems like effortless genius is actually the sum of many hours of hard work and practice that now lie deep inside the memory and support continued gains in performance.

Working to enhance your recall abilities may even make you smarter. Enhancing short-term memory may improve fluid intelligence, the ability to reason and solve problems independently of existing knowledge.[31] The connection between training to enhance retention and intellect is borne out by brain scans showing that the same regions of the brain that become active when engaging working memory are activated during problem-solving and reasoning exercises. Researchers at Temple University reported encouraging findings from a study in which participants in a four-week program to build their working-memory capacity also made gains in reading comprehension.[32]

Building one's ability to remember important information can be seen as a path to "constructing a proactive brain."[33] One key way to build memory is to expose the brain to new experiences. Brain scan studies show that "novelty stimulates activity not only in the memory centers of the hippocampus/medial temporal lobe but also in the dopamine-rich midbrain areas responsible for motivation and reward processing. Because dopamine can enhance learning, anything you consider unique gives your proactive neurocircuitry more ammunition."[34]

Achieving your goals will likely require learning and committing to memory new knowledge and skills. In our work with teachers and students, we have created useful strategies to aid in retention and recall across learning contexts. The CRAVE formula set out in our book *BrainSMART 60 Strategies to Increase Student Learning*[35] sets out attributes of a memorable lesson:

Curiosity: Committing something to memory needn't entail repetitive drills of random, disconnected facts. You are more likely to remember information that piques your curiosity and compels you to look for answers. In the classroom, teachers may introduce new topics with intriguing "teasers" that engage students' attention and desire to learn more.

Relevance: You are more likely to devote time and attention to learning something that matters to you or helps you achieve an important goal.

Asking questions: This is the first step to finding the answers you will commit to memory.

Variety: Changing up forms of practice can help hold attention, especially in an enriched environment that gives the brain lots of opportunities to explore and grow.

Emotion: Finding an emotional connection drives attention and retention. That's why scenes from a movie that make you laugh or cry are so much more memorable than a dry classroom lecture delivered in a monotone. Engaging your emotions as you practice and practicing with others with whom you have an emotional connection are two ways to help wire what you need to learn into long-term memory.

The CRAVE formula also illustrates a simple memory strategy—that of creating mnemonics to tie together related concepts and aid in recall. Just a few examples of other effective tools to build your "memory muscle" include:

Set it to music. Singing the ABCs is a near-universal example among American children of the usefulness of this strategy, but you can easily create your own "memory songs" by setting out information to a familiar tune or rap rhythm. Creating memory songs also may help you to think more deeply about the subject matter as you set important words to music.

Mix it up. Explore new information in a variety of ways, including hands-on activities. Instead of just reading about a historical event, write and produce a play about it or recreate the scene with a diorama. Instead of just telling students about different forms of matter, engage them in an experiment to turn water into ice and steam.

Share it. Teachers have shared with us many effective variations of learning together to aid in recall. When Texas teacher Diane Dahl's students are learning new spelling words, they may write them in sand or trace them with their fingers on a partner's back.

These ideas incorporate novelty and movement into repetition that makes practice more memorable.

As Beilock puts it, these kinds of strategies can free up working memory to keep learning new information and "can also be advantageous for performing under pressure, say in an important test or a do-or-die pitch to a client. ... Combining what you need to remember into meaningful wholes helps to ensure that some pieces don't get lost when it counts the most."[36]

A Personal Perspective on the Payoff for Hard Work

Through hard work and deliberate practice, we can even confront and set aside our fears. Public speaking ranks as a great fear among many people.[37] Marcus shares this personal story of how he overcame a terror of public speaking so great it caused him to stammer: I was a shy and quiet kid. I never felt I had much to add to the conversation, and when I did think of something to say, it often came out with a slight stutter. This inclination followed me into early adulthood when I found myself working on a project for an advertising agency in a professional development session at an Oxford University campus. For some reason, I volunteered to do the presentation for my team on a campaign to reduce truancy. I noticed that the presenters for other teams were creating support materials, writing prompt cards, and rehearsing. Having never before given a speech, I had no idea why they were doing this. I was busy with the team, brainstorming the strengths, weaknesses, opportunities, and threats of the challenge we had undertaken. The team was leaving it up to me to deliver the killer speech that would win us the prize and a probable boost to our careers.

Presentation day arrived. The panel of judges who would assess my performance consisted of a Who's Who of some of the most successful and creative people in the industry. The room was abuzz. As the rules for presentation were announced, I stood smiling and looking forward to my first speech. Following my introduction—"Let's have a round of applause for Marcus

Conyers presenting on behalf of his team"—I stepped to the podium and looked out at the judges and about 50 of my peers. My heart suddenly began to pound, my mouth went dry, and my mind completely blank. In that instant, I was transported back in time to my elementary classroom, where, caught daydreaming, I was ordered to the blackboard to write a word I could not spell. "Mr. Marcus Adrian Conyers, maybe you would like to come to the front of the class and spell the word *tomorrow*." (In my experience, nothing good has ever followed a parent or teacher using your full name.) More than a decade later, I could still smell the chalk dust and feel my hands begin to shake as I lifted the chalk hesitantly and heard the snickers of classmates behind me.

In a word, I "choked." The few words that I managed to deliver were rendered near-unintelligible by the return of my childhood stammer and followed by a booming, embarrassing silence. I was given an obligatory round of applause as I slumped down in my chair. The next presenter, someone I had seen days earlier doing strange things like writing prompt cards and rehearsing, was utterly brilliant. Later that day, one of the judges came up to me and said, "The applause you got was just like a Douglas Bader award." Bader was a British pilot in World War II who got shot down—a lot.

I could look at my first-ever presentation in one of three ways: (1) as a high-stakes gamble on my reputation among peers and potential future bosses, (2) as a complete disaster, or (3) as one of the most useful experiences of my life. I chose the third, reasoning that I had the potential to become a much better speaker. All I needed was to do the work to produce better results and to seek out new opportunities. I began reading everything I could on the topic. I asked businesspeople what they did to get ready for a presentation. Nothing really jelled. Then a colleague gave me a cassette tape about a completely different topic, the training of fighter pilots. The information was fascinating. Israeli pilots during the Six Day War shot down far more aircraft than the enemy. One reason was that they were mentally rehearsing positive outcomes. The thought struck me that I could do the same for presentations. I dubbed the thought process the "success simulator." To prepare for presentations, I would imagine effectively delivering a dynamic presentation, which helped me establish a positive and productive mindset.

The next boost to my presenting skills came after I moved to Toronto, Ontario, to run a small business. I arranged for a colleague and myself to be videotaped giving presentations so we could better assess our work. I soon learned a valuable lesson about the gap between my mind's-eye view of myself as a dynamic and engaging presenter and the truth captured on tape. My colleague wove a rich tapestry of fact and narrative, making his audience laugh and holding their attention. The camera captured a far different response from my audience—from yawns to outright dozing, furtive glances at watches, and restive feet tapping impatiently and pointed toward the door, yearning for escape. Eventually, even my copresenter nodded off briefly, and so did the camera operator, apparently, as the lens at one point drifted toward the ceiling before returning abruptly to the stage where I droned on. My colleague provided frank feedback about my sleep-inducing performance, which I realized was actually quite diplomatic when I viewed my presentation style for myself.

Back to research and reading I went. I discovered fascinating studies by Mehrabian indicating that only 7 percent of communication is verbal; the remaining 93 percent comes from voice tone and body language.[38] Eureka! I had the 7 percent down fine, just needed to work on the remaining 93 percent. I focused on voice inflection, facial expressions, and gestures, and I worked hard to convey the passion I felt for my message. I watched videos of great presenters and attended every presentation I could. To practice I delivered presentations on key topics at the Ontario Institute for Studies in Education for a national lecture organization. These presentations were open to the general public, so I got feedback from a diverse audience. Over time I came to love connecting to people by presenting. I was reading 200 books a year on learning, psychology, human performance, and emerging research on the brain. From this reading and research, I created frameworks and strategies for putting the research into practice. Every week,

I developed new material and refined my approach. Eventually, I was invited to present at a conference of the National Association of Elementary School Principals in Chicago, when I got my best evaluation results to date—and met my wonderful wife, Donna, the coauthor of this book.

My peers and judges at my first presentation would agree that I did not start out as a "natural" presenter. But I have improved, and I continue to work toward achieving more of my full potential in this arena. I have had the honor of giving keynotes in the United States and around the world, and I enjoy every minute of those presentations. Donna and I regularly present at educational conferences at the state, national, and international level. To continue to hone my presentation skills, I keep practicing and learning ways to "work smarter" through practical metacognition, the subject of the next chapter.

Notes

1   American Psychological Association. "Believing You Can Get Smarter Makes You Smarter." May 28, 2003. Retrieved from http://www.apa.org/research/action/smarter.aspx

2   Robert J. Sternberg. "Academic Intelligence Is Not Enough. WICS: An Expanded Model for Effective Practice in School and Later in Life." Paper commissioned for the Conference on Liberal Education and Effective Practice, March 12–13, 2009, p. 1. Retrieved from http://www.clarku.edu/aboutclark/pdfs/sternberg_wics.pdf

3   Sternberg, p. 6.

4   Geoffrey Colvin. "What It Takes to Be Great." *Fortune,* October 30, 2006. Retrieved from http://archive.fortune.com/magazines/fortune/fortune_archive/2006/10/30/8391794/index.htm

5   K. A. Ericsson, M. J. Prietula, and E. T. Cokely. "The Making of an Expert." *Harvard Business Review,* July–August 2007, p. 2. Retrieved from http://141.14.165.6/users/cokely/Ericsson_Preitula_&_Cokely_2007_HBR.pdf

6   Ericsson, Prietula, and Cokely, p. 3.

7   Ericsson, Prietula, and Cokely, p. 5.

8   K. A. Ericsson, R. T. Krampe, and C. Tesch-Romer. "The Role of Deliberate Practice in the Acquisition of Expert Performance." *Psychological Review,* *100*(3), 1993, p. 364.

9   Ericsson, Prietula, and Cokely, p. 5.

10 Bill Jensen. "The Biggest Distance in the World." In Michael Bungey Stanier (Ed.), *End Malaria*. The Domino Project, p. 91.

11 Jeff Brown and Mark Fenske. 2010. *The Winner's Brain: 8 Strategies Great Minds Use to Achieve Success*. Philadelphia, PA: Da Capo Press, p. 36.

12 Carole Ames and Jennifer Archer. "Achievement Goals in the Classroom: Students' Learning Strategies and Motivation Processes." *Journal of Educational Psychology, 80*, 1988, 260–267. Retrieved from http://www. unco.edu/cebs/psychology/kevinpugh/motivation_project/resources/ames_arc her88.pdf; Carol Dweck and E. L. Leggett. "A Social-Cognitive Approach to Motivation and Personality." *Psychological Review, 95*, 1988, 256–273.

13 Heidi Grant Halvorson. 2012. *Succeed: How We Can Reach Our Goals*. New York: Plume.

14 Grant Halvorson, p. 61.

15 Brown and Fenske, pp. 76–77.

16 Mihalyi Csikszentmihalyi. 1997. *Finding Flow: The Psychology of Engagement with Everyday Life*. New York: Basic Books, p. 27.

17 Csikszentmihalyi, p. 33.

18 Csikszentmihalyi, p. 117.

19 Roy F. Baumeister and John Tierney. 2011. *Willpower: Rediscovering the Greatest Human Strength*. New York: Penguin Press, p. 36.

20 Baumeister and Tierney, pp. 129–137.

21 Edward Hallowell. 2011. *Shine: Using Brain Science to Get the Best from Your People*. Boston: Harvard Review Press, p. 52.

22 Brown and Fenske, p. 39.

23 Baumeister and Tierney, p. 70.

24 "More Breaks May Help You Go with the 'Flow' at Work." Minds for Business: Psychological Science at Work, July 24, 2014. Retrieved from http://www.psychologicalscience.org/index.php/news/minds-business/more-breaks-may-help-you-go-with-the-flow-at-work.html

25 Angela L. Duckworth, Christopher Peterson, Michael D. Matthews, and Dennis R. Kelly. "Grit: Perseverance and Passion for Long-Term Goals." *Journal of Personality and Social Psychology, 92*(6), 2007, 1087.

26 Ibid.

27 Grant Halvorson, pp. 243–244.

28 Sian Beilock. 2010. *Choke: What the Secrets of the Brain Reveal About Getting It Right When You Have To*. New York: Free Press.

29 Richard Allington. 2009. *What Really Matters in Response to Intervention: Research-Based Designs*. Boston: Pearson Education.

30 Beilock, p. 56.

31 Sharon Begley. "Buff Your Brain: Want to Be Smarter in Work, Love, and Life?" *Newsweek*, January 9 and 16, 2012, pp. 28–35.

32 J. M. Chein and A. B. Morrison. "Expanding the Mind's Workspace: Training and Transfer Effects with a Complex Working Memory Span Task." *Psychonomic Bulletin & Review, 17*(2), 2010, 193–199. doi: 10.3758/PBR.17.2.193

33 Brown and Fenske, p. 127.

34 Brown and Fenske, p. 128.

35 Donna Wilson and Marcus Conyers. 2011. *BrainSMART 60 Strategies for Increasing Student Learning* (4th ed.). Orlando, FL: BrainSMART.

36 Beilock, p. 57.

37 Glenn Croston. "The Thing We Fear More than Death." *Psychology Today*, November 28, 2012. Retrieved from http://www.psychologytoday.com/blog/the-real-story-risk/201211/the-thing-we-fear-more-death

38 Albert Mehrabian. 1981. *Silent Messages: Implicit Communication of Emotions and Attitudes*. Belmont, CA: Wadsworth.

5

Working Smarter with Practical Metacognition

"Insight into our own thoughts, or metacognition, is key to high achievement in all domains."

—Stephen M. Fleming[1]

Metacognition may be seen as a foundation for learning, achievement, and success in almost any field.[2] In our work in teacher education, many educators have told us that the cognitive and metacognitive strategies they've taught to their students have also made a positive difference in their professional practice and personal lives. Traditionally, metacognition has been defined as "thinking about your thinking." We propose a model that goes beyond thinking to action. We define *practical metacognition* as the process of establishing clear intent about what we want to achieve; planning and executing action steps; and assessing, monitoring, and adjusting our thoughts and actions so that we keep making progress.[3] Using practical metacognition can help you become positively smarter in many ways, such as enabling you to identify your strengths and deploy them to achieve your goals and to recognize potential limitations and self-correct when needed.

Positively Smarter: Science and Strategies for Increasing Happiness, Achievement, and Well-Being, First Edition. Marcus Conyers and Donna Wilson.
© 2015 John Wiley & Sons, Inc. Published 2015 by John Wiley & Sons, Inc.

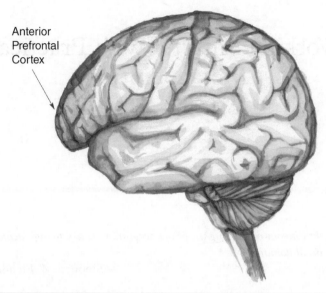

Anterior
Prefrontal
Cortex

Figure 5.1 The Area of the Brain Associated with Metacognition.
© 2015 BrainSMART, Inc.

Neuroscientists are now making headway in discovering the centers of metacognition in the brain. A team of researchers at University College London reported that subjects who demonstrated higher levels of metacognition had more gray matter in the anterior prefrontal cortex and more white matter (which facilitates the transmission of electrical impulses across neurons) connecting the anterior prefrontal cortex to other parts of the brain (Figure 5.1). The researchers acknowledge that more studies are needed to determine how the anterior prefrontal cortex supports metacognition, but suggest that "these findings are a crucial first step toward identifying ways to shore up metacognition, whose absence can produce devastating effects."[4]

Thus far, we have discussed how practical metacognition and the cognitive skills under its umbrella contribute to making the most of neuroplasticity, achieving greater happiness, maintaining a positive outlook, and putting in the work to achieve one's goals. In this chapter, practical metacognition takes center stage. By developing this ability, we become attuned to wielding the thinking, problem-solving, and interpersonal strategies we need to acquire and improve our knowledge and skills. We make gains each day at applying these strategies, reviewing our progress, and figuring out whether and how we need to adjust our thinking. We consciously consider and become better at answering key questions, such as:

- What do I need to learn to accomplish my goals?
- What strategies will help me learn the necessary knowledge and skills most effectively?
- How does this new knowledge fit in with what I already know?
- How will I know if my developing knowledge and skills are up to the task?
- How can I best translate my effort and practice into long-term results?
- Can I apply this new knowledge or skill in other situations?

One of our all-time favorite reactions to learning about metacognition is that of a Texas third grader, who recognized that learning to think about her thinking would make her "the boss of my brain." Donna's practice as an educator was transformed when she began to discover how the use of metacognitive tools can make the difference between student success and failure. For example, I remember how guiding a middle schooler to use metacognition to stop and think before starting a fight kept him from another suspension. His father thought it was the magic bullet! In another instance, a high school student learned how to consciously slow down and make better decisions about the organization of her research projects instead of starting impulsively and then turning papers in without editing responsibly.

For adults, developing cognitive and metacognitive skills can help you "grapple and grow," *Shine* author Edward Hallowell notes, so that "the hard work is also smart work, that effort is leading to growth."[5] Applying the cognitive and metacognitive strategies set out in this and other chapters can indeed help you work smarter and take advantage of the 80/20 principle—capitalizing on the 20 percent of effort and practice that account for 80 percent of results!

Among the cognitive and metacognitive concepts we have presented thus far are selective attention to stay focused on positive progress; the CIA strategy of recognizing and optimizing where you have control and influence and accepting where you do not to make the most of your opportunities; and strategies to strengthen memory and translate the results of practice into long-term memory. This chapter introduces a framework for employing these strategies throughout the learning process and highlights additional strategies to guide you on your path to becoming positively smarter. Table 5.1 provides an action assessment of

Table 5.1 Action Assessment: Employing Cognitive Assets to Work Smarter

On a daily basis, how often do you ...	Almost never	Sometimes	Frequently	Consistently
1. Establish your clear intent.				
2. Proceed with appropriate courage through the steps you need to accomplish your goals.				
3. Engage in systematic planning and searches for the information you need to work smarter.				
4. Manage your time wisely.				
5. Accurately assess situations and adjust your thoughts and actions accordingly.				

(continued)

Table 5.1 Action Assessment: Employing Cognitive Assets to Work Smarter (*cont'd*)

On a daily basis, how often do you ...	*Almost never*	*Sometimes*	*Frequently*	*Consistently*
6. Learn from experience.				
7. Finish what you start.				

key cognitive assets. How many of these strategies are in your metacognitive toolkit?

The Input–Processing–Output Model of Learning

Learning is not an isolated event but a process. In each phase of that process, you can take actions that will improve how and what you learn and lead to better long-term gains applying your new knowledge and skills. The conceptualization of learning as *information processing*[6] is structured around four central concepts:

1. Thinking involves perceiving and encoding external stimuli (what we see and hear and do in interacting with other people and our environment) into memory.
2. We analyze and store those encoded stimuli to enable future decision making.
3. We then draw on these stored memories to handle similar situations in the future, modifying this stored data when necessary.
4. Our thinking continues to expand and evolve as we apply our base of information in problem solving and decision making on an ongoing basis.

Applying this information processing model, we developed an approach to learning and teaching called *Thinking for*

Results, which divides the process of learning into three major phases:[7]

Input. You identify your learning goals—what new skills you will need to develop, what information you will need to gather and where you can find it, and what additional support you may need in the form of special lessons, coaching, and practice. In effect, you develop your plan for learning.

Processing. In this phase, you gather the information, study and analyze it, and connect it with what you already know. You learn and practice new skills. This second phase is what most people think of as "learning." Oftentimes, you will link back to the first phase as you discover new paths of learning—things you didn't realize at the beginning that you will need to learn to achieve your goals. You revise and expand your learning plan and gather additional information for processing and practice.

Output. Finally, you demonstrate your newly formed knowledge and skills and apply them in a variety of situations. In the classroom, the output phase takes the form of written papers, science projects and demonstrations, classroom presentations, and tests and other forms of assessment. Outside formal education, examples of output might include using a new computer language you've learned to write a program, speaking a new language you've learned as you travel, harvesting a garden after trying some new planting and maintenance techniques, and improving your run times after developing your stamina with a cross-training regimen.

It is helpful to view learning through this three-phase model because you can more easily identify breakdowns and obstacles to achieving your goals and take corrective action. For example, if you really want to learn a new language but you're having a hard time, you can step back and analyze each phase.

- **Input:** Do you have the best resources for learning? Is there a different course, online outlet, or teacher that might help improve your learning?

- **Processing:** Are you devoting adequate time to studying and practicing the language? Are there specific areas of learning, such as speaking vs. reading vs. understanding when others speak, where you need to devote more effort?
- **Output:** Do you have an effective feedback component in testing your developing language skills? Would it be helpful to interact with someone who is fluent in the language to provide practical direction about areas where you may need additional practice and suggestions for additional resources to take your language learning to the next level?

In this way, you can come to see learning not as an isolated task, but as an ongoing process in which you are continually building on what you know and setting new goals. Learning becomes a way of life, an integral undertaking to becoming ever more positively smarter!

Cognitive Assets You Can Develop to Work Smarter

Within the input–processing–output phases of our Thinking for Results model are a range of *cognitive assets* that support practical metacognition. These strategies and abilities can be used at all phases of learning and share in common these factors:[8]

- **Cognitive assets are not personality traits.** That is, they are not innate attributes of what make you unique (though they can make you stand out!). They are learnable and teachable, and the more you use them, the better results you will realize.
- **Cognitive assets are useful in all aspects of your life,** in both your personal and professional pursuits.
- **People from all walks of life and at the full range of current abilities will benefit from learning to use cognitive assets.** They are useful to craftspeople, academics, health care providers, hospitality workers, musicians and artists,

programmers and developers, entrepreneurs, and retired people pursuing their favorite hobbies.

- **The use of cognitive assets can help support a positive outlook.** And, conversely, maintaining a positive outlook can help you make the most out of your cognitive assets.
- **Cognitive assets can help you pursue what you care most deeply about,** and in doing so, build knowledge and skills in an incremental, stepwise approach. As you become more knowledgeable and skilled in one area, those gains carry over into other aspects of your life and improve your confidence and optimism in undertaking future challenges.

In short, cognitive assets are the tools in your practical metacognition toolbox, which you should keep by your side ready for use at home, at work, and in all your personal endeavors.

Clear Intent[9]

At the heart of accomplishing your goals is developing your clear intent. Knowing what you want is the first step to getting it. Clear intent provides the roadmap for purposeful living and a motivational touchstone to keep you moving in the right direction. Identifying your clear intent makes it easier for you to use the rest of the cognitive assets presented here as effectively as possible.

To zero in on your clear intent, consider these questions:

- What do I want?
- Why do I want it?
- When do I want it?
- How will I know when I have achieved it?
- Does this goal lead me to a greater mission, and if so, what is that mission?

Clear intent can propel us to action at the individual level ("I want to eat healthier and get more exercise"), at the family or small group level ("We want to include more fruits and vegetables in our meals and reduce empty calories"), and in communities and beyond. In the early 1960s, when President Kennedy shared his goal of sending a man to the moon and safely home again and accomplishing that ambitious undertaking within a decade, he was modeling clear intent. Achieving that goal entailed a huge commitment of resources and setbacks and heartache along the way, but clear intent kept the nation behind it.

Appropriate Courage[10]

People demonstrate appropriate courage when they are willing to commit to the new experiences that are necessary to achieve their aims. This strategy involves accurately assessing the risks of an endeavor to ensure that it is consistent with your mission and goals—and then taking the next step. As Dr. Robert Biswas-Diener notes in his essay "Stop Complaining and Muster the Courage to Lead":

> Courage is simply acting in a way that puts you at risk in a fearful or uncomfortable situation in which the outcome is uncertain. Sticking up for an underdog at a team meeting is an act of courage. Launching a new product is an act of courage. Confronting a supervisor on a point of disagreement is an act of courage.[11]

An example of appropriate courage might be signing up for a course to learn a necessary new skill and then actively participating in the course to get the most it has to offer and to internalize what you are learning toward your own aims. Or it might involve organizing a noontime workout group to motivate yourself and coworkers to achieve shared fitness goals. Taking these kinds of actions may require that you step out of your comfort zone by speaking out in a room full of strangers or trying something new, but they are necessary to accomplish your ultimate aim. Appropriate courage involves an accurate assessment of three Rs:

- What **results** do I want?

- What are the **rewards** of pursuing this opportunity?
- What are the **risks** involved in this opportunity?

Systematic Search and Planning[12]

For many people, achieving their full potential will require them to proactively hone their organizational skills. A lucky few may seem "naturally organized"; the rest of us have to work at it. We define the cognitive strategies of systematic search and planning as appropriate exploratory and planning behavior that is organized to lead to an intended and well-expressed response. Systematic search, the purposeful identification and gathering of information necessary for learning, embodies the essence of the input phase, and systematic planning entails an active approach for putting this learning to use. These questions are at the center of systematic search and planning:

- What goal do you want to accomplish? As with many cognitive assets, systematic search and planning are rooted in your clear intent.
- What are useful sources of information to help achieve this goal? For example, if you want to improve your eating habits, you might conduct an Internet search on healthy food choices, find resources at the library, consult your physician, and talk with a nutritionist.
- Are these sources of information credible and useful for your purposes? In assessing credibility, consider the knowledge base of the person or organization supplying the information, the intent of making this information available (to make money? to entertain? to share important data or to purposefully lead people astray?), and the support for this information from other sources.
- Once you have collected the necessary information, what do you need to do to put it to best use? What steps will you need to take to accomplish that aim?
- What resources will you need to accomplish your plan?
- What is your time frame to complete your plan?

Understanding and Managing Time[13]

Hand in hand with systematic planning goes the ability to effectively budget the time necessary to bring a plan to fruition. As with organizational skills, some people seem to have well-calibrated internal clocks and allocate their time efficiently, meet deadlines, and arrive on time for appointments. These attributes are typically the products of good habits developed over time rather than some innate ability. This means that even if you feel your sense of time is out of whack with that of the rest of the universe, you can still develop your time management skills and use them in support of achieving your goals, such as improving your work performance and earning a promotion or making the time to learn a new skill.

How people think about time may have a cultural component. For example, promptness may be measured in minutes or hours. Your understanding of time must be in sync with the demands and expectations of your work and personal life—whatever those demands and expectations may be.

At one point in his career, Marcus managed communications for an international airline with offices in 30-plus countries. The culture of an airline requires being on time. If people are late, then planes are late, and planes make money by flying reliably on time. That culture taught me a useful strategy about how to make sure to be on time:

1. Double check the start time of classes, meetings, and appointments.
2. Plan to arrive at least 10 minutes early.
3. Determine how long it will take you to get where you need to be.
4. Write down your departure time.
5. Leave at your departure time, whatever else happens.

This strategy can be adapted for other purposes, such as estimating and scheduling time needed to accomplish crucial tasks and pacing yourself to accomplish timed tasks such as tests and physical workouts.

Cognitive Flexibility[14]

Another example of a strategy that is especially crucial to achieving your potential is cognitive flexibility, or the skill and capacity for accurately assessing situations and adjusting your thoughts and actions appropriately. Flexibility is a hallmark of creative thinking and problem solving. If you are confronted by a problem that seems unsolvable, it is often helpful to back up and assess your basic assumptions about the problem, to seek out and consider differing points of view about it, and to try out new ideas and approaches. Developing cognitive flexibility requires you to be open to new ideas, to the perspectives of others, and to the possibility that there may be better ways to do things.

In opposition to cognitive flexibility is the mindset that there is only one "right way" to do things and that the best way to accomplish a task is to do it the way you've always done it. In the business arena, successful companies value innovation and continual improvements in their products and processes. To accomplish these aims, their employees must be flexible thinkers, always on the lookout for new and better ideas.

Along the same lines, on the way to achieving your full potential, you will encounter many existing obstacles and new challenges. Developing your cognitive flexibility can help you deal with those roadblocks. Consider these guiding questions:

- Is what I am currently thinking and doing the best way to accomplish the goals I have set for myself?
- What are my cues for assessing my progress?
- If things are not going as well as they might, what do I need to do differently and how can I think differently?

We are strong advocates that living life to the fullest in the 21st century requires embracing lifelong learning. We live in an age of information and innovation. To thrive in the workplace, we must be ready and willing to adapt to new technologies and processes, many of which carry over into our personal lives as well. Cognitive flexibility—the willingness to consider new ideas and different ways of thinking and doing—is a key aspect of lifelong learning, of continually striving to achieve your potential.

Learning from Experience[15]

Embrace your mistakes as the great learning experiences that they are. A fundamental aspect of a positive classroom environment is that students are encouraged to take intellectual risks and to look on mistakes as opportunities to correct and improve their learning. The same is true for adults pursuing learning goals: Recognizing that you don't understand something or that there may be a better way can be a giant step forward. For example, recurring problems at work are a signal that you need to evaluate the systems and processes involved for possible improvements. If you experience a setback in your personal endeavors, such as plateauing in your fitness regimen or harvesting a lower-than-expected yield from your garden, you may want to consult a print resource or expert on changing your approach. Learning is often a trial-and-error process, and progress comes from recognizing both mistakes and successes and from correcting one and building on the other:

- What went wrong?
- What are some of the possible causes of this problem?
- What are some possible solutions, and how can I test each of them to figure out which one is the best path?
- How can I avoid this problem in the future?
- What went right?
- Is there a way to do it even better?

Finishing Power[16]

Finishing power entails effective task completion sustained over time and in spite of difficulty to accomplish essential goals. Two guidelines are at the core of finishing power:

- Finish what you start.
- Start only what you intend to finish.

We recall the story of a gifted young girl who loved to write. She filled notebooks with fantastic stories—which no one ever read. Sometimes a story remained unfinished because she didn't come up with an ending; more often the author refused to share her stories because they "needed more work." But instead of going back and editing the first drafts she had already written into a form she considered ready for publication, she turned her attention to writing new stories.

This vignette exemplifies two tendencies that stand in the way of finishing power. Some people tend to start projects with enormous energy, but as their enthusiasm wanes, they either get distracted by other endeavors or they finish projects halfheartedly. Other people may fall victim to perfectionism, unable to let go of a project until it is "perfect"—and since few things in life are perfect, they are never done.

To facilitate finishing power, consider these guiding questions:

- Why is it important to complete this task?
- What will it feel like when you celebrate completing this task?
- What obstacles do you need to anticipate and overcome to complete this task?
- How long will it take to accomplish this task, and how can you schedule the time to do so?
- What steps do you need to take to complete this task?

As you can see, the cognitive strategy of finishing power is related to other assets, including systematic planning and understanding time. And as with other assets, it involves maintaining a focus on your clear intent to finish what you start and purposeful action. Finishing power requires clearly envisioning at the beginning of a task what you need to do to accomplish it, how you will know when you are done, and what you will gain by successfully completing it.

Pacing on the Path to Positively Smarter

Many people who have succeeded in becoming positively smarter rely on these kinds of cognitive strategies, perhaps without naming or consciously applying them. A proactive approach to applying practical metacognition can help you work smarter. Especially if there is a gap between your goals and your achievement, you may benefit from thinking through how you use your cognitive assets through the stages of input, processing, and output to more successfully achieve your aims.

Even if you have developed every possible cognitive strategy, you will need to pace your learning and set realistic goals to maximize your potential. As Hallowell notes, "You can't sprint to peak performance." He goes on to explain:

> While a computer can work all day and all night, a brain cannot. It needs rest, food, human engagement, and stimulation. It must be managed with care. If you sprint—work flat-out—for too long, your brain will deplete the neurotransmitters and other neurochemicals required to sustain top performance. We often forget that *thinking is work*. It requires energy, which is in finite supply and must be replenished regularly. To think well, the brain requires oxygen, glucose, and a host of nutrients and other factors, all of which get depleted over time. Without the right diet, sleep, exercise, and physical supports (good lighting, air supply, chair and desk, and so on), the brain will underperform.[17]

In Chapters 7 and 8, we will explore these imperatives in more detail by examining the role of improving your physical well-being in becoming positively smarter. As Table 5.2 shows, achieving your cognitive potential to optimize your optimistic outlook, neuroplasticity, and productivity relies on your abilities to wield the cognitive assets set out throughout this text, to use your cognitive space effectively, and to keep your cognitive fuel tank full.

Table 5.2 Powering up Your Practical Metacognition

Component	Description	How to "power it up"
Cognitive potential	The capacity to learn knowledge, skills, and attitudes needed to achieve success in school, career, and life.	Maintain a positive outlook about your ability to succeed through hard work, learning, and practice.
Cognitive assets	Skills and abilities to facilitate input, process, and output knowledge to improve problem solving, creativity, collaboration, and communication.	Learn to use these assets in your daily life and work on improving them through conscious practice over time.
Cognitive space	The short-term capacity we use for handling events as they happen; also known as working memory.	Focus your selective attention on one task at a time to improve performance; multitasking may clog up cognitive space (see Chapter 3). Practice and memory strategies can help make some tasks more automatic and less cognitively demanding (see Chapter 4).
Cognitive fuel	Factors that fuel the brain for performance.	Exercise regularly to improve oxygen and blood flow and to refocus when attention is lagging. Eat nutritious foods, with a balance of lean protein, complex carbohydrates, unsaturated fats, and vitamins, minerals, and nutrients from fruits and vegetables (see Chapters 7 and 8).

Practical Metacognition in Action: Lessons from the Grameen Bank

Concerned about the high rates of poverty in his homeland, Bangladesh, economics professor Muhammad Yunus led his students on a research project in the village of Jobra. They interviewed local women who were struggling to support their families by weaving and selling bamboo furniture; by the time they had repaid the high interest to moneylenders on loans to buy supplies, they made just pennies in profit. Unable to find a bank willing to lend to the weavers at fair rates, Yunus loaned 42 women a total of $27 as seed money for their enterprise. That small investment allowed them to launch their business successfully and repay the loans with interest. Based on that experience, Yunus formed Grameen Bank, which means Village Bank, to make microloans to independent craftspeople and business owners too poor to qualify for financing from traditional banks. Grameen Bank and its customers have thrived—with a repayment rate higher than 97 percent—and Yunus and his bank were awarded the Nobel Peace Prize in 2006 for efforts "to create economic and social development from below."[18]

One valuable lesson that Yunus learned from this work is that "each of us has much more hidden inside us than we have had a chance to explore. Unless we create an environment that enables us to discover the limits of our potential, we will never know what we have inside of us."[19] What we find so moving and relevant about this story is how it captures the essence of maintaining an optimistic outlook that positive change is possible through the application of creative solutions supported by metacognition. Yunus and his students developed their clear intent to create a new financial model to support the weavers of Jobra and their appropriate courage to make fairly priced loans to the villagers. They displayed cognitive flexibility in thinking about banking in a new way and executed systematic planning, time management, and learning from experience in creating Grameen Bank from this experiment in a single village. And their finishing power is evident in the fact that Grameen has become a model for micro-lending enterprises to combat poverty in many countries.

The story of Muhammad Yunus and the weavers of Jobra also illustrates another key element of becoming positively smarter—the gains that are possible when we work and learn together. In the next chapter, we explore our "social brains," how the inter-reliance of ancient people working and hunting together may have influenced the evolution of human brain development that endowed our species with the neuroanatomy for collaboration, teamwork, and greater social capital.

Notes

1 Stephen M. Fleming. "The Power of Reflection: Insight into Our Own Thoughts, or Metacognition, Is Key to Higher Achievement in All Domains." *Scientific American*, September/October 2014, p. 31.

2 Fleming, p. 32.

3 Donna Wilson and Marcus Conyers. "The Boss of My Brain." *Educational Leadership*, 72(2), October 2014. Retrieved from http://www.ascd.org/publications/educational-leadership/oct14/vol72/num02/%C2%A3The-Boss-of-My-Brain%C2%A3.aspx; Donna Wilson and Marcus Conyers. 2011. *Thinking for Results: Strategies for Increasing Student Achievement by as Much as 30 Percent* (4th ed.). Orlando, FL: BrainSMART.

4 Fleming, p. 35.

5 Edward M. Hallowell. 2011. *Shine: Using Brain Science to Get the Best from Your People*. Boston: Harvard Business Review Press, p. 136.

6 Robert Sternberg. 1987. "Information Processing." In R. L. Gregory (Ed.), *The Oxford Companion to the Mind*. New York: Oxford University Press.

7 Wilson and Conyers, *Thinking for Results*.

8 Wilson and Conyers, *Thinking for Results*, pp. 123–125.

9 Wilson and Conyers, *Thinking for Results*, pp. 145–147.

10 Wilson and Conyers, *Thinking for Results*, pp. 224–226.

11 Robert Biswas-Diener. "Stop Complaining and Muster the Courage to Lead." In Michael Bungey Stanier (Ed.), *End Malaria*. The Domino Project, p. 115.

12 Wilson and Conyers, *Thinking for Results*, pp. 154–156; 188–190.

13 Wilson and Conyers, *Thinking for Results*, pp. 169–171.

14 Wilson and Conyers, *Thinking for Results*, pp. 191–193.

15 Wilson and Conyers, *Thinking for Results*, pp. 231–232.

16   Wilson and Conyers, *Thinking for Results*, pp. 227–230.
17   Hallowell, p. 33.
18   Nobelprize.org. Retrieved from http://www.nobelprize.org/nobel_prizes/ peace/laureates/2006/press.html
19   Grameen Bank Web site, Preface by Muhammad Yunus. Retrieved from http://www.grameen.com/index.php?option=com_content&task=view&id= 211&Itemid=380

6

Better Together

"Increasing evidence suggests that one of the primary drivers behind our brains becoming enlarged was to facilitate our social skills—our ability to interact and get along well with others."

—Matthew Lieberman[1]

The human brain stands apart in the animal world—three times the size of our nearest primate relative[2] and 50 percent greater in proportion to body size than the next nearest animal (the bottlenose dolphin).[3] We aren't the fastest animals on the planet or the strongest; the longstanding assumption for why we are the brainiest centered on our analytical skills, problem-solving abilities, and capacity for abstract thought. Then in the early 1990s, anthropologist Robin Dunbar published an article in the *Journal of Human Evolution*, reporting on his research comparing the size of the neocortex in relation to the rest of the brain in humans to that of other primates based on the size of the social group on which each species relies and interacts with regularly. For example, the neocortex-to-brain ratio of a Tamarin monkey is about 2:3, and its "tribe" typically numbers about 5; a Macaque monkey has a brain size ratio of about 3:8 and a social group of around 40. Given the

Positively Smarter: Science and Strategies for Increasing Happiness, Achievement, and Well-Being, First Edition. Marcus Conyers and Donna Wilson.
© 2015 John Wiley & Sons, Inc. Published 2015 by John Wiley & Sons, Inc.

much larger size of the human neocortex in relation to the rest of
the brain, Dunbar extrapolated that our brains evolved to become
much larger in order to manage the complex interrelationships of
a social group numbering about 150.[4] This "social brain hypothesis" is consistent with anthropological and historical data across
almost 8,000 years, from 6000 BC well into the 18th century, that
humans settled in villages with consistently around 150 others.[5]
This seems to be the optimal population for bringing together
a "clan"—again, this is Dunbar's terminology—of sufficient but
not overwhelming numbers for hunting, gathering, and supporting each other. In other words, evolution might have favored early
humans with bigger brains who survived because they were able
to navigate the personal interactions of hunting in groups for big
game rather than fighting over a rabbit for dinner! As Dunbar and
colleagues note in a later article: "The underlying assumption is
that the neocortex provides the computational power to manage
the complex web of social relationships needed to give a social
group its cohesion and stability through time."[6] These findings
remain highly relevant in modern society, Matthew Lieberman
suggests in his book *Social*:

> Each of us needs to navigate complex social networks to be success-
> ful in our personal and our professional lives. Primate brains have
> gotten larger in order to have more brain tissue devoted to solv-
> ing these social problems, so that we can reap the benefits of group
> living while limiting the costs.[7]

This is an astonishing shift in thinking about human brain
development—from assuming our species developed big brains to
power analytical acumen to finding evidence that what separates
us from other animals is, more than any other factor, our social
nature and the size of our social networks. There has been an
explosion of research on social cognition and brain development in
recent years. In fact, the Social and Affective Neuroscience Society
(SANS) was founded in 2008 to bring together research investigat-
ing the neural basis of social and affective (or emotional) processes.

The emerging field of interpersonal neurobiology focuses on the brain as a social organ adapted throughout life by its owner's experiences; in other words, scientists in this realm study how the social parts of our brain develop as a result of experience-dependent plasticity.[8]

Dunbar and his colleagues have continued to lead the way in studying how social interactions relate to the structure and functioning of the brain. Twenty years after the introduction of the social brain hypothesis, their latest iteration of research investigates the impact of social functioning at the individual level. The researchers compared the social network size (personal contacts or communications in the previous seven days), social cognitive competency (as measured by a test of *Theory of Mind*, the ability to assess the intentions and mental states of other people), and volume of the orbital prefrontal cortex (the area of the brain associated with social information, planning, language, and memory processing) of 40 participants. The study offered two crucial conclusions: "The relationship between brain size and social group size applies not just between species, but even at the level of the individual within species," and "this relationship is mediated by social cognitive abilities."[9] It appears that people with the biggest brains (at least the greatest volume of gray matter in their orbital prefrontal cortex) may not be the smartest people in the room, but they certainly have the best-developed social abilities!

Thus, scientists are uncovering evidence that neuroplasticity—the idea that "practice makes cortex"—applies not only to analytical skills but also to our social competence, our ability to interact in positive and productive ways with family, friends, colleagues, and others. This emerging field of research, an important new area of educational neuroscience, has exciting implications for personal development and relationships, for education, and for workplace productivity. Specifically for our purposes, it appears that learning, working, and playing with others can bolster our quest to become positively smarter. How many of the strategies in Table 6.1 do you use in your daily interactions with others?

Table 6.1 Action Assessment: Honing Your Social Intelligence

On a daily basis, how often do you ...	*Almost never*	*Sometimes*	*Frequently*	*Consistently*
1. Accentuate the positive in your interactions with others.				
2. Listen effectively.				
3. Carefully consider others' points of view.				
4. Consciously establish rapport.				
5. Take advantage of opportunities to learn with others.				
6. Encourage and support others.				
7. Participate actively in and contribute to your many "communities."				

Born to Be Social: Impact on Health and Well-Being

From infancy on, human beings rely on each other, and social connections are vital to our well-being. What babies need most, Lieberman notes, is caregivers who are committed to providing for their needs. Of course, infants need food, water, and shelter, but because they cannot obtain these necessities for themselves, their most fundamental requirement is for a caregiver to provide for them. "Love and belonging might seem like a convenience we can live without, but our biology is built to thirst for connection because it is linked to our most basic survival needs."[10] And because brain development in the early years is so intensive, the care and attention that infants receive from their parents and other regular caregivers has a disproportionate impact on their neural development.[11]

Throughout life, the correlation between social connections and physical health persists. Positive personal relationships appear to provide a protective effect down to the molecular level of body functions, facilitating the production of cells that strengthen our immune systems and slowing processes associated with aging, Cozolino writes. "Social support not only provides direct salubrious effects on mind and body but also buffers us against the negative effects of stress. ... For example, being around supportive others reduces blood pressure, stress hormone levels, autonomic and cardiovascular reactivity, and the risk of illness."[12] Maintaining social connections has been shown to support cardiovascular health, general health status, and mental health, including a lower incidence of depression and anxiety and better emotional regulation than people who spend a great deal of time in isolation. In fact, one conclusion of a review of more than 100 medical studies is that people who have risk factors for developing health problems and who maintain extensive social connections are less likely to become ill than people with the same risk factors who are more isolated socially.[13]

Regular, positive social interactions are also associated with less severe cognitive decline in older adults and greater longevity. A variety of studies show that "those with more types of relationships—for example, being married; having close family members, friends, and neighbors; and belonging to social, political, and religious groups—live longer."[14]

Social well-being is one of three essential components of mental health, along with emotional and psychological well-being, according to a classification system for assessing mental health.[15] One of the authors of that system, Corey Keyes, identified five dimensions of social well-being: social acceptance, the extent to which we maintain positive attitudes toward others; social actualization, our belief that together we can make the world a better place; social contribution, our belief that our daily activities contribute to and are valued in our communities; social coherence, our ability to make sense of society; and social integration, whether we feel that we are a part of a community where we are supported and support others.[16]

Anatomy of the Social Brain

The inner workings of our social brain are evident in the ways our facial expressions and mannerisms reflect those of the people near us, often unconsciously. Donna provides a few personal examples: At one point when we were working together on this book, I had a break-through about a difficult passage, and as I was explaining it to Marcus, I saw his face break out in the same big smile I knew I was wearing. Along the same lines, I came across a photo of my niece Anna and me taking a stroll, with the length of our strides and the positions of our bodies in uncanny unison. Marcus also tells me that when I go into "teaching mode," he notices that my head lifts and my face moves forward—which I recall as the pose of a favorite teacher and colleague of mine.

These natural tendencies to imitate others may result from the firing of *mirror neurons*, special cells that are activated when we see others taking an action with familiar intentions. In his book *Mindsight*, Daniel Siegel explains that mirror neurons are at work in the simplest and most complex of human interactions. From birth, our brains begin to store information about the sequences and patterns of others' actions and emotions that allow us to understand and respond in kind to their intentions. "We sense not only what action is coming next, but also the emotional energy that underlies the behavior."[17] Siegel describes the connections between the mirror neuron systems in the frontal and parietal lobes of the cortex through a neural structure called the *insula* to the limbic system and brainstem, sending the signals that direct our facial expressions, movements, and even heart and respiratory rates, as the "resonance circuits ... the pathway that connects us to one another."[18]

141

Neuroscientists continue to study the extent to which mirror neurons and/or other structures in the brain are responsible for our earliest learning. Researchers conducting experiments with newborns report that infants respond to and mimic the actions of their parents and other adults within hours and days of birth. The mimicry may begin with sticking out their tongues but ultimately extends to such complexities as motor skills and the cadence and regional accent of speech. This research suggests that "a wide range of behaviors—from tool use to social customs—are passed from one generation to another through imitative learning."[19]

Other research has identified areas in the frontal and parietal lobes of the cortex as becoming active during *mentalizing,* or applying one's Theory of Mind (see the discussion in the following section). It is intriguing that these areas coincide with the brain's default system, the regions that are most active when we think we are not thinking about much at all.[20] When our brains are not engaged in conscious cognitive tasks, they tend to gravitate toward thinking about people—ourselves and others. Lieberman suggests that this reflexive tendency to reflect on the social aspects of our lives "promotes understanding and empathy, cooperation, and consideration. It suggests that evolution, figuratively speaking, made a big bet on the importance of developing and using our social intelligence for the overall success of our species by focusing the brain's free time on it."[21]

Throughout life, we become fully ourselves within our social worlds as a part of the brain's amazing plasticity, especially experience-dependent synaptogenesis. Starting with our earliest attachments to our parents and other caregivers, our social world is at the center of our map of who we are. Thanks to the marvelous plasticity of the hippocampus, the brain structure that is key in the development of conscious memories from about age three onward, we are able to consciously create memories of our lives with others across the life span. Through connections between the limbic center, the prefrontal cortex, and other regions of the brain, we are continuously in the process of becoming!

Getting "Socially Smarter"

Taken together, this diverse research suggests a strong connection between maintaining supportive social networks and becoming positively smarter: By developing and maintaining our social competence, we can enhance the quality and quantity of our relationships, both personal and professional. And by extending our social networks, we also continually enhance our social competence—providing yet another example of the upward spiral that can increase our happiness, productivity, and well-being.

Psychologists and social scientists studying the realm of interpersonal relationships define *social cognition* as our knowledge about interacting with people and the way we think and reason about those interactions. A fundamental aspect of social cognition is referred to as *Theory of Mind,* an understanding that each person has beliefs, desires, knowledge, and intentions and that other people's mental states are different from ours. Most people develop Theory of Mind over time from early childhood, though autism appears to impair the ability to develop this social understanding. Kindergartners typically are aware that it is possible to imagine events that are not real and that each person has feelings that may be different from their own. These understandings become increasingly sophisticated, especially with guidance from parents and teachers, as children learn to recognize that they and others may have conflicting emotions and motivations and that the best way to resolve an argument may be to consider an issue from the other person's perspective.

For example, a group of European researchers examined whether training school-age children to recognize the emotions of people they read about enhanced their social cognition. With one group of children, the researchers read illustrated scenarios and led discussions about how the characters felt and how their emotions influenced their actions. Another group of students read the same stories and were asked to draw a picture about them, with no discussion. The training group performed better than the control group on assessments of comprehending emotions and responding empathetically—that is, seeing things from the other

143

people's point of view and reflecting their emotional responses—and these gains in social understanding persisted over the several months of the study.[22]

Another example of developing Theory of Mind comes not from humans, but from a clever chimp in an African forest. Every morning the chimp and the rest of its group traversed the same path searching for food. Researchers who had set up cameras to record the chimps' comings and goings set a single banana along the path. The next morning, the first chimp spied the banana, paused, and then let out a howl as if it had spied a snake. The other chimps quickly scampered up trees, while the first chimp sat down to a nice breakfast. The chimp had employed Theory of Mind to comprehend what would cause the other animals to scatter so it could have the banana all to itself.[23]

As with developing an optimistic outlook and enhancing your knowledge and skills, it is possible to improve your social cognition—not to devious ends like that crafty chimp but to enjoy more positive relationships in your personal life and more productive interactions in the workplace. In fact, many of the strategies presented in earlier chapters can also support the development of your social intelligence. Let's consider a few key strategies and their application at home, in the classroom, and on the job.

Accentuate the Positive

Put simply, happiness springs from being with people whose company you enjoy, and people prefer to be around happy people. Recognizing and appreciating the positive attributes of the people in your life enhances your relationships. Modeling an optimistic outlook and offering positive encouragement brings out the best in you and the people in your life. In fact, "happiness spreads throughout social networks up to three degrees of separation. That is, if you are happy, this can impact your friend and your friend's friend as well."[24]

Having studied the interactions of married couples for years, John Gottman and Julie Schwartz Gottman can tell within minutes of meeting a couple and observing their interactions whether their marriage is likely to last.[25] Among the principles that reinforce the positive aspects of marriage and help these unions endure through tough times is the need to proactively develop a positive view of your spouse and to know and encourage his or her hopes and interests. The Gottmans have even quantified the ratio of positive to negative (characterized by criticism and contempt) communications: People in stable, supportive marriages shared five positive remarks for every negative remark when discussing a conflict; in comparison, couples whose marriage ultimately ended in divorce shared less than one positive statement for every negative remark to or about each other. This research underscores that positive encouragement is especially crucial when the going gets tough. When you have people who care about you offering their support, you are more likely to persist through challenges to achieve your aims.

Sharing a positive outlook is also crucial in education. As we have noted previously, children are more likely to thrive academically in positive classroom and school environments where they feel safe, secure, accepted by teachers and peers, and encouraged to take intellectual risks. Guiding students to maintain an optimistic outlook enhances the likelihood that they will persist in learning tasks until they succeed. Sharing stories of optimism in action can help illustrate the gains that are possible when you believe you can succeed. Nevada kindergarten teacher Christena Nelson illustrates the power of a positive approach in a puppet show featuring Tess the Treasure Hunter, who always looks on the bright side and believes that she and her friends will succeed if they keep trying and encourage each other, and Grumpy Gus, who sees rain in every cloud and is easily discouraged. When she asks her students whether they want to be more like Tess or Gus, they clamor, "We're Tess! We're Tess!"

Setting a positive tone does not require elaborate preparation. In workshops, we have found that offering healthy snacks or a simple gift such as an inspirational quote on an index card at the start of the session can set the tone for a positive experience. At some events where we have presented, the sponsoring organizations have used music as a mood enhancer as participants enter the room where we are delivering keynotes.

Polish Your Listening Skills

Becoming an effective listener is at the center of enhancing your social relationships. Learning to direct your selective attention to listening carefully to others will enhance other social cognition abilities, such as understanding others' perspectives and building rapport. Many teachers who guide their students to learn and use the HEAR strategy[26] tell us that it helps to focus students' attention on learning and improve their interactions with others. You may realize these benefits as well, when you follow these steps to become a better listener:

Halt: Stop whatever else you are doing, end your internal dialogue on other thoughts, and free your mind to pay attention to the person speaking.

Engage: Focus on the speaker. It may help to adopt a physical component, such as turning your head slightly so that your right ear is toward the speaker, as a reminder to engage solely in listening.

Anticipate: Look forward to what the speaker has to say. By anticipating his or her message, you ensure that your attention is focused on the speaker. This step also aids in remembering the message.

Replay: Think about what the speaker is saying. Analyze and paraphrase it in your mind or in discussion with the speaker and others. Replaying the information will aid in understanding and remembering what you have learned.

Good listening skills are essential in the business world—for providing the best possible customer service and complaint resolution, for building trust and heading off conflict among coworkers, and for leaders to understand what is happening in their organizations and to maintain positive momentum and motivation. The ability to listen well is among the top skills employers seek in job candidates, notes communications professor Andrew Wolvin. "Effective listening is recognized as key to organizational success because poor listening can be costly."[27]

Consider Others' Points of View

Closely linked with effective listening is the ability to consider other people's points of view. Developing this skill begins with the recognition that other people hold beliefs and perspectives that may differ from yours and that they have (or believe they have) valid reasons for doing so.[28] This ability is facilitated by curiosity and respect for others and an openness to consider new ideas. As the writer F. Scott Fitzgerald wrote, "The test of a first-rate intelligence is the ability to hold two opposed ideas in the mind at the same time and still retain the ability to function."[29]

To consider other people's points of view, begin by listening without judging or immediately filtering or blocking with your own beliefs what others are saying. If you are building an opposing response in your mind while the person is speaking, you are not listening effectively. Ask questions to clarify if anything seems unclear and paraphrase what the speaker has said to ensure your understanding. Only then should you compare the message with your beliefs and perspectives. After hearing and considering others' points of view, you may find that you have learned something new and interesting—a different way of looking at the world. You may discover that your perspectives are not so different than the speaker's and that what you have in common forms a strong basis for continued discussion, reflection, and learning. Or you may decide that the message is in conflict with your beliefs and knowledge you will continue to hold, but at least you have listened with respect and civility and considered what the other person has to say.

Making the effort to understand other people's points of view can fulfill a very human need. "Much of human behavior is driven by the need to belong and the desire to connect with others," write three California researchers who conducted an experiment with UCLA students on their physiological reactions to "feeling understood" and not understood.[30] "The results demonstrated that feeling understood activated neural regions previously associated with reward and social connection ... while not feeling understood activated neural regions previously associated with negative affect."[31] The differences between feeling understood or not also activated different components of the brain's mentalizing system. The study charts how our emotional responses coincide with the brain's processing as we seek to forge a connection of understanding with others.

To find an example of the pitfalls of a failure to make the effort of understanding others' points of view, we need only to look at the gridlock in Congress. Too many elected officials from both parties are far more interested in scoring political points with their "base"—voters in their districts and states who mirror their views—than in working together to solve problems. That proclivity to shout others down rather than listen may begin in our nation's capital and work its way down to the electorate, or legislators may believe they are simply reflecting their constituencies' insistence not to compromise on certain issues. Either way, it seems to have brought us to a continual impasse that is unproductive at best and dangerous at worst. In response to this highly charged political climate, the National Institute for Civil Discourse was formed to promote the need for considering and respecting others' points of view. Chaired by former presidents representing both major parties, George H. W. Bush and Bill Clinton, the institute is conducting research and advocacy with the mission of "fostering an open exchange of ideas and expression of values that will lead to better problem-solving and more effective government."[32] We propose a bottom-up approach to help replace the current counterproductive, vitriolic style of governing: If each of us is more open to considering others' points of view at home, in school, and in the workplace, the world will be a much better place for it.

Establish Rapport

In Chapter 4, we described the pleasant and productive state of being in flow. The equivalent of finding flow in social relationships might be in establishing rapport. As with the state of flow, developing rapport through empathetic interactions with others produces positive cognitive and physiological responses. Think back to an interaction you've had with others in which you felt in total harmony. You might have been working on a home or work project together, playing a game, enjoying a concert, or absorbed in deep conversation. In his book *The Brain and Emotional Intelligence*, Daniel Goleman notes that "these moments of interpersonal chemistry, or simpatico, are when things happen at their best."[33] The "physiology of rapport" entails three components: paying full attention to one another, becoming physically in synch to the point of adopting the same gestures and facial expressions, and sharing positive feelings.

Rapport sometimes occurs naturally, but you can also consciously direct your mind and actions to develop these connections with others. For example, taking the time to convey empathy and getting to know the colleagues you are working with in teams can help to make those relationships more constructive and beneficial and further the positive climate in your workplace. Goleman suggests that it is possible to develop the "core skill" of empathy, which takes three forms: cognitive empathy ("I know how you see things; I can take your perspective"), emotional empathy (which he describes as "the basis for rapport and chemistry"), and empathic concern ("I sense you need some help and I spontaneously am ready to give it").[34] From these descriptions, it is easy to see how conveying an empathetic approach might enhance your relationships with family, friends, colleagues, and others. When you are able to develop sincere, positive connections with others, they are more likely to accept your encouragement and support and to listen to your ideas—and to provide the same support and encouragement when you need it.

Learn Together

Yet another benefit of positive social relationships is that we can often be more creative and productive together than individually. This "better together" dynamic is evident in findings about the academic gains that students can make when they learn from each other. Social learning, or collaboration in pairs, small groups, and whole classes, has been found to boost achievement as children share what they know and expand their knowledge by comparing their perspectives and learning strategies with others. Peer tutoring may enhance learning for both the tutor and the student receiving guidance: The tutor has to think deeply about the lesson content to teach it, and the other student gains from learning with a person who is the same age and may present the material quite differently than the teacher and the text. As educational researcher John Hattie notes, "when students become teachers of others, they learn as much as those they are teaching."[35]

Social learning works for adults, too. When we have opportunities to learn through collaboration, we gain insights from others' experiences and expertise and can share our own, and everyone's learning experience is richer for that exchange. Donna recalls some good advice from her first meeting with cognitive psychologist Reuven Feuerstein: It was 1989. I had read his book *Instrumental Enrichment*[36] and was applying many of its principles in my work as a school psychologist. I was also thinking that what I really wanted to do was to move into teacher education, to share effective approaches to classroom instruction with other educators. But I wondered if I was up to this challenge, and I confessed my qualms when I met Professor Feuerstein following a presentation. He just took my hand and asked if I knew what a ricochet was. Then, he said gently in his lilting accent, "Donna, as you teach it, you will better learn it. It will come back to you!" This has proven to be so true. When we present at conferences and professional development sessions, I learn a great deal from the questions and comments of participants as they share how the concepts we are teaching apply to their professional practice.

Become a Great Encourager

Realizing your goals to become positively smarter becomes a lot easier when you have the support and encouragement of caring others—and the people in your social networks are more likely to reciprocate when you make a habit of offering encouraging words. "Just ask people who regularly achieve peak performance what the key to their success is," Hallowell suggests. "Like happy people, most often they will tell you about a person—a parent, a coach, a teacher, a partner, a spouse, a manager early in their careers—who believed in them and drew out of them more than they knew they had. That's the magical power in connection."[37]

Encouragement may take many forms, from the whole-hearted support of parents, to the caring guidance of teachers, to the exacting standards and reinforcement through practice with coaches and instructors, to the role models provided by mentors and bosses in the working world. It is supplied by spouses who nudge their husbands and wives on to pursue their dreams and sometimes even make accommodations in family life to make those pursuits possible. It can be found in siblings, grandparents, and friends who are there to cheer for successes and talk through challenges and setbacks. American culture values the iconic image of strong individuals making it on their own, but in reality, most everyone who succeeds in achieving their aims has had someone in their corner to lend support in some form or another.

Educational research suggests that encouragement is most effective when it is specific and individual and emphasizes effort and process over praise for achievement. For example, parents and teachers can share with children the clear message that they have what it takes to achieve their learning potential and that fulfilling their dreams will require hard work and persistence. The most effective way to support children's progress in school and in other endeavors is to focus on the value of their effort, not just on results such as grades on tests, ribbons for 4-H projects, or trophies for sports and dance competitions.

Praising children for their effort rather than focusing on achievement shines the spotlight on their learning gains and the importance of hard work and persistence that lead ultimately to mastery of new knowledge and skills. This form of encouragement sends the message that mistakes are part of learning and that it's OK to take on ambitious goals that will likely entail some setbacks along the way. Recognizing children as the unique individuals they are and for their positive attributes also enhances their good feelings about themselves.[38]

Contribute to the "Social Capital" of Your Community

These strategies for enhancing social connection function at the individual level but also have implications for communities. You likely belong to several "communities"—of colleagues at work, immediate and extended family, circles of friends, peers in school, teammates and enthusiasts with shared athletic interests, fellow hobbyists and participants of leisure-time activities, neighbors, and members of fraternal and civic organizations, church congregations, and other associations. By applying the abilities and strategies discussed in this chapter, you can contribute to the *social capital* of your communities, doing your part to strengthen the network of relationships among people for the betterment of all. As community activist, educator, and author Cecile Andrews notes, developing empathy with others is the best way to effect positive change: "You can't get people to change by loading them up with facts or shaking your finger at them. You must talk to others with respect and caring—and then you connect. Social capital is thus central to progressive social change."[39]

Social capital emphasizes the "we" rather than the "I," without sacrificing individuality. This form of capital grows through shared trust and information, cooperation, and the reciprocity of people helping people and knowing they can rely on the same kind of help when they are in need. Just as financial capital grows through the accumulation of earnings, social capital is enhanced by the willing contributions of a community. Compton and Hoffman summarize the research in this area: "When a society has a high level of social capital, then there is a greater sense of trust in other people, more reciprocity and helpfulness, greater participation in social and civic activities, and stronger social ties."[40]

Ultimately, the degree to which neighbors and citizens support each other and work together to successfully solve their community's problems may determine the extent to which the community exhibits learned powerlessness or learned empowerment. The latter is demonstrated through a sense of *collective efficacy*, or "social cohesion in a community that creates local friendship networks and a sense of agency, or a willingness to intervene in making one's neighborhood a better place to live."[41]

That dynamic can bolster communities defined by geography and by other attributes, including businesses and institutions whose success relies on the positive and productive interactions of their employees and members. As just one example, a school's climate is a reflection of the outlook of students, teachers, and administrators. Is there a shared belief and optimism that all students have the potential to excel? Do teachers believe they have the capacity to make a positive difference in their students' learning? Do administrators and teachers collaborate with a shared focus on students' academic success?

Each member of a community contributes to its social capital, but leaders, whether they hold formal or informal titles to leadership, play an especially crucial role in setting the tone for how well people interact and support each other. A recent business study surveyed employees about the most important attributes of leaders. Five of the top seven leadership skills involved bringing out the best in people: inspiring and motivating others, displaying high integrity and honesty, communicating powerfully and prolifically, collaborating and promoting teamwork, and building relationships.[42] The message is clear: The ability to lead a team or organization in which people work well with others at all levels is critical for productivity and success.

Being Social in a High-Tech World

It is a pleasure and privilege to lead our teams at BrainSMART and the Center for Innovative Education and Prevention. We have the honor of working in the realm of teacher education with a group of people who are committed to the mission of supporting effective teaching so that all children receive a high-quality education that prepares them for the challenges and opportunities of life in the 21st century. The team has been working together for many years and has now developed a great deal of trust. Each of us realizes that we are not good at everything, nor are we good alone. Each of us has strengths we amplify together. As leaders we surround ourselves with teammates who can do well what we can't. The story of our work together attests to the power of the social brain. We are a virtual team spread across North America in a half-dozen states and a Canadian province, but the same attributes of successful collaboration apply—respect, trust, open communications, acknowledgment of each other's strengths and contributions, and support for each other.

The teachers who study in the graduate degree programs offered through Nova Southeastern University also are distributed across the continent and throughout the world. Some mention in surveys that they had a few qualms about an online program before enrolling, but the vast majority quickly come to appreciate the virtual discussions and the ease with which they can share and receive feedback from their professors and far-flung peers. Like us, these teachers are excited to be able to connect with other people who are passionate about education. We enjoy continuing productive online conversations with these educators and with colleagues we've met at professional conferences. Online communities have helped teachers break out of the isolation of their classrooms and share effective teaching strategies with peers in their districts and states, across the country, and around the world.

In addition, we love sharing and seeing photos of family and friends and following their pursuits and adventures via Facebook, and it is wonderful to be able to chat on Skype. We can stay connected with folks in Donna's hometown in Oklahoma and Marcus's in England and with family and all the friends we've made through the years no matter where they have settled or how far they roam.

Early studies on the impact of the "information superhighway" on its users' human connections, released in the late 1990s, were discouraging, pointing to increased isolation and withdrawal from friends and family. But over time, cyberspace has yielded to our social natures and become a common tool to connect with others.[43] Social networks like Facebook, Twitter, and Pinterest are helping to bring people together, whether they are across the hall in a college dormitory or across oceans. Ten years after its founding in 2004, Facebook had signed on 1.32 *billion* members in its online global community, with an average 829 million signing on daily.[44] "Because Facebook use is more of an extension of real-world connections, it has been associated with enhancing offline social networks and general well-being. It's also particularly useful for maintaining social bonds over long distances," Lieberman notes. "We should make use of these ways of connecting or savoring connections because they make us happier and healthier."[45]

In short, engaging our social brains can make us happier, more productive, and healthier in person and online. In the next two chapters, we turn to the well-being component of becoming positively smarter as we explore how regular exercise and healthy nutrition support optimal functioning of our bodies and brains.

Notes

1   Matthew D. Lieberman. 2013. *Social: Why Our Brains Are Wired to Connect.* New York: Crown, p. 28.
2   Esther Herrmann, Josep Call, María Victoria Hernàndez-Lloreda, Brian Hare, and Michael Tomasello. "Humans Have Evolved Specialized Skills of Social Cognition: The Cultural Intelligence Hypothesis," *Science, 317*(5843), September 7, 2006, 1360–1366. Retrieved from http://www.sciencemag.org/content/317/5843/1360.full
3   Lieberman, p. 29.
4   R. I. M. Dunbar. "Neocortex Size as a Constraint on Group Size in Primates." *Journal of Human Evolution, 22*(6), June 1992, 469–493; Michael Harré. "Social Network Size Linked to Brain Size." *Scientific American,* August 7, 2012. Retrieved from http://www.scientific-american.com/article/social-network-size-linked-brain-size/
5   Lieberman, p. 32.
6   Joanne Powell, Penelope Lewis, Neil Roberts, Marta Garcia-Fiñana, and R. I. M. Dunbar. "Orbital Prefrontal Cortex Volume Predicts Social Network Size: An Imaging Study of Individual Differences in Humans." *Proceedings of the Royal Society B: Biological Sciences,* February 1, 2012. Retrieved from

http://rspb.royalsocietypublishing.org/content/early/2012/01/27/rspb.2011.
2574.full

7   Lieberman, p. 35.

8   Louis Cozolino. 2014. *The Neuroscience of Human Relationships: Attachment and the Developing Social Brain* (2nd ed.). New York: Norton, p. xvii.

9   Powell, Lewis, Roberts, Garcia-Fiñana, and Dunbar.

10 Lieberman, p. 43.

11 Cozolino, p. xvii.

12 Cozolino, p. 244.

13 Leonard Mlodinow. "The Importance of Being Social." Guest Blog on *Scientific American* Streams of Consciousness Blog, April 24, 2012. Retrieved from http://blogs.scientificamerican.com/streams-of-consciousness/2012/04/24/the-importance-of-being-social/

14 Sheldon Cohen and Denise Janicki-Deverts. "Can We Improve Our Physical Health by Altering Our Social Networks?" *Perspectives on Psychological Science*, 4(4), 375–378. Retrieved from http://www.ncbi.nlm.nih.gov/pms/articles/PMC2744289/

15 Corey L. M. Keyes and Shane Lopez. 2002. "Toward a Science of Mental Health: Positive Directions in Diagnosis and Interventions." In C. R. Snyder and S. Lopez (Eds.), *Handbook of Positive Psychology* (pp. 45–59). London: Oxford University Press.

16 Corey L. M. Keyes. "Social Well-Being." *Social Psychology Quarterly*, 61(2), June 1998, 121–140.

17 Daniel J. Siegel. 2010. *Mindsight: The New Science of Personal Transformation*. New York: Bantam, p. 61.

18 Siegel, p. 60.

19 Andrew N. Meltzoff. 2005. "Imitation and Other Minds: The 'Like Me' Hypothesis." In S. Hurley and N. Chater (Eds.), *Perspectives on Imitation: From Neuroscience to Social Science* (Vol. 2, pp. 55–77). Cambridge, MA: MIT Press. Retrieved from http://web.cs.swarthmore.edu/~meeden/DevelopmentalRobotics/05Meltzoff_Like_Me_Hypth.pdf

20 G. L. Shulman, J. A. Fiez, M. Corbetta, R. L. Buckner, and colleagues. "Common Blood Flow Changes Across Visual Tasks II: Decreases in Cerebral Cortex." *Journal of Cognitive Neuroscience*, 9, 1997, 648–663.

21 Lieberman, pp. 19–20.

22 Veronica Ornaghi, Jens Brockmeier, and Ilaria Grazzani. "Enhancing Social Cognition by Training Children in Emotion Comprehension: A Primary School Study." *Journal of Experimental Child Psychology*, 119, 2014, 26–39. Retrieved from http://www.academia.edu/4966555/Enhancing_social_cognition_by_training_children_in_emotion_comprehension_A_primary_school_study

23 Cozolino, p. 371.

24 William C. Compton and Edward Hoffman. 2013. *Positive Psychology: The Science of Happiness and Flourishing* (2nd ed.). Belmont, CA: Wadsworth, p. 271.

25 John M. Gottman and Julie Schwartz Gottman. 2006. *10 Lessons to Transform Your Marriage*. New York: Crown.

26 Donna Wilson and Marcus Conyers. 2011. *BrainSMART 60 Strategies for Increasing Student Learning* (4th ed.). Orlando, FL: BrainSMART, p. 281.

27 Andrew D. Wolvin. 2009. "Listening, Understanding, and Misunderstanding." *21st Century Communication: A Reference Handbook*. Thousand Oaks, CA: Sage. Retrieved from Sage Reference Online, http://www.sagepub.com/edwards/study/materials/reference/77593_5.1ref.pdf

28 Donna Wilson and Marcus Conyers. 2011. *Thinking for Results: Strategies for Increasing Student Achievement by as Much as 30 Percent* (4th ed.). Orlando, FL: BrainSMART, p. 217.

29 F. Scott Fitzgerald, "The Crack-Up," *Esquire*, February 1936. Available online at http://www.esquire.com/features/the-crack-up

30 Sylvia A. Morelli, Jared B. Torre, and Naomi I. Eisenberger. "The Neural Bases of Feeling Understood and Not Understood." *Social Cognitive and Affective Neuroscience* Advance Access, January 5, 2014, p. 2. Retrieved from http://sanlab.psych.ucla.edu/papers_files/Morelli(2014)SCAN.pdf

31 Morelli, Torre, and Eisenberger, p. 1.

32 National Institute for Civil Discourse, "Mission." Retrieved from http://nicd.arizona.edu/purpose

33 Daniel Goleman. 2011. *The Brain and Emotional Intelligence: New Insights*. Northampton, MA: More Than Sound, p. 57.

34 Goleman, p. 61.

35 John Hattie. 2009. *Visible Learning: A Synthesis of Over 800 Meta-Analyses Relating to Achievement*. New York: Routledge, p. 187.

36 Reuven Feuerstein, Yaacov Rand, Mildred B. Hoffman, and Ronald Miller. 1980. *Instructional Enrichment: An Intervention Program for Cognitive Modifiability*. Baltimore, MD: University Park Press.

37 Edward M. Hallowell. 2011. *Shine: Using Brain Science to Get the Best from Your People*. Boston: Harvard Business Review Press, p. 81.

38 Donna Wilson and Marcus Conyers. 2013. *Flourishing in the First Five Years: Connecting Implications from Mind, Brain, and Education Research to the Development of Young Children*. Lanham, MD: Rowman & Littlefield Education, p. 108.

39 "Social Ties Are Good for Your Health," interview with Cecile Andrews. BeWell@Stanford, undated. Retrieved from https://bewell.stanford.edu/features/social-ties-good-health

40 Compton and Hoffman, p. 270.

41 Compton and Hoffman, p. 272.

42   Jack Zenger and Joseph Folkman. "The Skills Leaders Need at Every Level." *Harvard Business Review* HBR Blog Network, July 30, 2014. Retrieved from http://blogs.hbr.org/2014/07/the-skills-leaders-need-at-every-level/

43   Lieberman, p. 255.

44   Facebook Newsroom. Retrieved August 18, 2014, from http://newsroom.fb.com/company-info/

45   Lieberman, p. 256.

7

Building a Smarter Body–Brain System Through Exercise

"The whole brain flourishes as a result of movement. It provides the environment that brain cells need to grow and function well."
—John Ratey and Richard Manning[1]

An active body is a healthier body, and exercise has tremendous benefits for the brain as well. The final component in our mission to become positively smarter is to improve our physical well-being through regular exercise, sleep, and nutrition. As the research and recommendations set out in this chapter will demonstrate, the benefits of regular aerobic exercise and strength training accrue not only to physical health but to enhanced brain functioning as well, a compelling example of neurocognitive synergy in action:

- Regular physical activity is associated with a larger hippocampus, a brain area involved in memory and spatial processing, and bolsters brain regions in charge of executive function.
- It increases the production of the brain chemical BDNF, referred to as "effective fertilizer for the brain,"[2] and supports the production of new neurons and synapses.

Positively Smarter: Science and Strategies for Increasing Happiness, Achievement, and Well-Being, First Edition. Marcus Conyers and Donna Wilson.
© 2015 John Wiley & Sons, Inc. Published 2015 by John Wiley & Sons, Inc.

- It increases angiogenesis, the growth of blood vessels that improve oxygen flow to the brain.
- Exercise can help reduce symptoms of depression.
- It is an excellent stress buster and puts us in a more positive mood, which in turn can make us more creative and productive.
- Improved physical health enhances happiness and feelings of subjective well-being.

Regular physical activity benefits people of all ages. Incorporating movement and exercise into the school day enhances academic achievement and starts young people off on the right path to a daily routine that includes physical activity. Older adults who exercise regularly enjoy greater health and sharper minds. Many of the aspects of aging—including muscle mass, strength, basal metabolic rate, body fat percentage, aerobic capacity, blood-sugar tolerance, cholesterol levels, blood pressure, bone density, and internal temperature regulation—are within our control, suggest medical researchers William Evans and Irwin Rosenberg. Whatever the current level of fitness, regular exercise, encompassing both aerobic and strength training, "is the prime mover in the drive to preserve vitality," especially when combined with good nutrition (the subject of our next chapter):

> You do have a second chance to right the wrongs you've committed against your body. Your body can be rejuvenated. You can regain vigor, vitality, muscular strength, and aerobic endurance you thought were gone forever. ... This is possible whether you're middle-aged or pushing 80. The "markers" of biological aging can be more than altered: in this case of specific physiological functions, they can actually be reversed.[3]

We refer to the *Body–Brain System* to emphasize how the interconnections of cognition, emotions, and our physical selves influence our readiness, motivation, and ability to learn and to thrive.[4] After reviewing the research on the role of exercise in enhancing well-being, we will present helpful guidelines on incorporating physical activity into your daily routine. According to the Centers for Disease Control and Prevention, only 20 percent of American adults are currently doing the amounts of aerobic exercise and strength training recommended to maintain healthy bodies and brains,[5] so most of us will benefit from following these guidelines! Complete the action assessment in Table 7.1 on your current level of physical activity.

Table 7.1 Action Assessment: Working Out Your Body–Brain System

In a typical week, how often do you ...	1–3 times	4–6 times	Daily	Total time (in minutes)
1. Engage in aerobic exercise that raises your heart and respiratory rate.				
2. Engage in strength training that works out all your major muscle groups.				

Work Out the Body to Keep the Brain Young

Losing mental acuity is one of the most common worries of older adults.[6] The good news is that exercise can keep your brain nimble—without having to invest in an expensive gym membership or wait for years to reap the benefits of your workouts. Research shows that a brisk walk or other aerobic exercise several times a week is a brain-healthy habit that can begin to pay off in weeks rather than months or years.

Some regions of the brain may shrink as we age; for example, some studies show the hippocampus loses from 0.5 percent to 2 percent of its mass annually after age 50, which is associated with memory impairment and cognitive difficulties over time.[7]

To assess whether physical activity might reverse or slow this trend, researchers at the University of Illinois recruited healthy adults ages 55 to 80 who didn't exercise regularly and divided them into two teams; one group walked 40 minutes three days per week and the other performed stretching and balance exercises during the trial period. Participants in the study underwent MRI scans to measure the volume of their hippocampi before, during, and after this period. Among participants in the walking team, the size of their hippocampi increased an average 2 percent, while those in the stretching and balance group experienced an average decrease of 1 percent. This research suggests that (1) a moderate regimen of physical activity may counteract some of the effects of aging on the brain and (2) it's never too late to begin to realize these benefits.[8]

Another group of researchers reported similar results, indicating that "aerobic exercise training is effective at reversing hippocampal volume loss in late adulthood, which is accompanied by improved memory function."[9] And a third study concluded that "even shorter term aerobic exercise can facilitate neuroplasticity to reduce both the biological and cognitive consequences of aging to benefit brain health in sedentary adults."[10] These researchers evaluated changes in brain blood flow, cognition, and fitness in 37 subjects ages 57 to 75 who engaged in one-hour aerobic workouts three times a week for 12 weeks. Compared to a control group, the study participants showed increased blood flow in their hippocampal regions, improved performance on tests of immediate and delayed memory, and increased physical stamina.

Regular physical activity also may help to enhance optimism and control mood disorders. Routine exercise has been shown to increase activation in the left hemisphere of the brain, which supports a more positive outlook, and to reduce right hemispheric activity associated with stress and negative thinking.[11] Research connecting regular exercise to the alleviation of depression goes back more than three decades. In one study with three groups of subjects diagnosed with depression, one group of people took part in an aerobic exercise program, a second group took Zoloft, and a third did both. After 16 weeks, symptoms of depression had eased in participants in all three groups, which suggests that exercise may be as effective as medication—and perhaps more so over the long term. In a follow-up study, participants from all three groups who exercised regularly were less likely to relapse. Another study focusing on frequency of exercise found that people who walked fast for about 35 minutes a day five times a week or 60 minutes a day three times a week reported a lessening of their mild to moderate depression symptoms; in comparison, walking fast for 15 minutes a day five times a week or doing stretching exercises three times a week did not help as much.[12] The positive impact of exercise on depression may be related to the release of endorphins or the neurochemical norepinephrine.

Regular aerobic exercise supports better blood flow and oxygen intake throughout the body and brain, which enhances our stamina for both physical and mental workouts. One study found that a brisk 30-minute walk five times a week stimulates production of BDNF, which facilitates both neurogenesis and synaptogenesis.[13] In recent years, scientists have also identified a hormone induced by aerobic exercise, called irisin, that may help burn calories more efficiently and increase the expression of BDNF.[14] In short, research suggests that regular aerobic exercise supports a healthier, happier, bigger brain!

New Muscle Is Young Muscle

Picture someone lifting weights and what do you see in your mind's eye? The stereotype might be a young male training for football or getting in shape for a beach vacation. However, new understandings about the power of strength training suggest that men and women of all ages can benefit from this activity. In fact, no matter what your age, strength training can help you become healthier and stronger and can improve your cognitive functioning as well. "If you rest you rust," warns physician Karl Knopf in his book *Weights for 50+*. "People who do not engage in a regular strength-training routine will lose 40 to 50% of their muscle mass and 50% of their muscular strength by age 65."[15]

Adding muscle contributes to "vitality of your whole physiological apparatus," note Evans and Rosenberg.[16] Because each pound of muscle burns calories much more efficiently than a pound of fat, improving the body's muscle-to-fat ratio helps to increase your metabolic rate; enhances aerobic capacity and overall cardiovascular health; triggers muscles to use more insulin, which reduces the risk of developing diabetes; and helps to maintain higher levels of HDL, or "good cholesterol." In other words, as we add muscle, we build a better fat-burning engine that keeps burning more calories, even at rest.

To the conventional wisdom that middle-aged and older adults should focus on aerobic exercise and ignore weight lifting, physician Bob Arnot counters that "muscle is youth. ... Muscle is completely rebuilt at least several times per year. So even at age eighty, well-trained muscle is really young."[17] In effect, strength training as one part of a healthy lifestyle may actually turn back the biological clock 10 to 20 years: "A healthy active person ages approximately half a percent a year compared to an inactive person with poor health habits who ages at approximately two percent a year."[18]

Obviously, then, the sooner you incorporate strength training into your physical fitness regimen, the better. Research from Tufts University suggests that health improvements are possible whenever you begin. In the study, 12 people ages 60 to 72 were encouraged to train three days a week for 12 weeks under the watchful eyes of the researchers. The amount of weight the participants lifted increased every week as they got stronger. At the end of the study, both a scan of muscle mass and a muscle biopsy to assess progress at the cellular level supported the already-obvious results of the tri-weekly workouts: Older adults can expect to add as much muscle growth as younger people doing the same amount of exercise.[19] In fact, many of the participants in the Tufts study were able to lift more weight than the 25-year-old graduate students who were working with them in the laboratory. This research is a tremendous addition to what we are learning about the potential for human beings to stay strong as we age.

Another study was conducted at the Hebrew Rehabilitation Center for the Aged, which is a chronic care hospital. This time, the study group consisted of 10 men and women ranging in age from 87 to 96 years old. The focus of this research was somewhat different, with the aim of establishing the relationship between participants' muscle strength and how long it would take them to walk 20 feet. Walking time was established as a functional way to measure leg strength. In the eight-week study, the researchers found that even frail, institutionalized elderly people could build strength through exercise. The leg muscle strength of participants almost tripled, and the size of their thigh muscles increased by 10 percent. One of the participants, a 93-year-old man, said, "I feel as though I was 50 again. The program gave me strength I didn't have before. Every day I feel better, more optimistic."[20]

Evidence that strength training supports brain health as well is supplied by research from the University of British Columbia: Women exhibiting symptoms of early dementia were divided into groups to compare the efficacy of cardio exercise and weight training on their cognitive functions. Only participants who did weight training showed significant improvements in both memory and executive functions. Brain scans supported these findings, indicating increased neural activity following weight training. Lead researcher Teresa Liu-Ambrose reported, "The take-home message is that even if you are beginning to see signs of cognitive impairment, the brain is still capable of rebounding with the right kind of physical activity. Weight training, even as little as once or twice a week, can minimize the rate of cognitive decline and change the disease course."[21]

From these studies, we can see that our physical potential persists throughout the life span and is both a matter of the brain and the body. We can also see in the words of one of the study's participants the interconnection of brain and body power. Building body strength had the added benefit for these older adults of instilling a sense of accomplishment and optimism that they can do whatever they set out to do. That is the very definition of becoming positively smarter.

The Body–Brain System Inside and Outside the Classroom

Of course, the benefits of regular physical activity on cognitive functioning are not limited to older adults. As many teachers can attest, incorporating exercise into the school day can help students focus on learning, and research continues to explore how moving their bodies benefits young brains. In one of many studies reported in recent years, Swedish medical researchers connected a heart-healthy diet and exercise to improved school performance for teenagers and young adults.[22] Along the same lines, a 2002 study of fifth, seventh, and ninth graders in California found a "consistent positive relationship between overall fitness and overall achievement." The author of that study, James Grissom, cautioned that physical fitness did not automatically result in academic gains; rather, "it is more likely that physical and mental processes influence each other in ways that are still being understood."[23]

Aiding in that understanding is research from Dartmouth professor Michele Tine on the impact of aerobic exercise on the academic performance of children and adolescents. Just 12 minutes of exercise improved students' selective visual attention and reading comprehension, and those improvements were stronger for students from low-income households than peers from higher socioeconomic backgrounds.[24] Tine suggests the difference in performance based on income levels might be related to stress; disadvantaged students are more likely to be coping with chronic stress, which has been shown to interfere with learning. Because exercise is an effective stress management tool, physical activity for these students may offer an additional benefit.

The Body–Brain System has many applications in education to support students' academic potential. Regular physical activity and incorporating movement, music, and art into lessons engage the body and brain in productive ways. In its report on *Health and Academic Achievement,* the Centers for Disease Control and Prevention lists a variety of benefits from incorporating exercise, even short activity breaks of 5 to 10 minutes, into the school day: improved cognitive performance, increased academic achievement, better attendance, and more positive, on-task behavior.[25] We have long championed physical education, music, and art as core subjects alongside math, science, English, and social studies. Students' active participation in these classes and activities, dismissed in some school districts as expendable as they seek to deal with budget shortfalls, supports learning in all subjects.

The experience of the Naperville Community Unit School District 203 in suburban Chicago is particularly instructive. Since requiring daily physical education for all students as part of its "culture of fitness," Naperville schools have posted significant gains on standardized tests. The school district continues to study how to make the most of this connection between physical activity and academic performance. One strategy has been for struggling high schoolers to take phys ed right before their most challenging classes; at Central High School students who took phys ed directly before English read on average a half year ahead of those who didn't and students who took PE right before math posted big gains in standardized tests, according to a PBS report.[26] Naperville schools have been recognized by the Centers for Disease Control and Prevention for their commitment to encourage students to be fit for life.

Beyond this direct connection between body and brain fitness, incorporating movement in the school day supports learning in several ways by:

- **Enhancing attention.** When students' attention begins to wander, teachers report the benefits of short exercise or stretching breaks or an active recess on the playground in helping to resharpen the focus on learning.
- **Building creative, motor, and social skills through play.** "Play is the most creative activity of the human brain. In play the brain totally lights up," notes author Edward Hallowell.[27] For young children especially, active play enhances motor skills such as object control (throwing and catching), coordination, balance, and hand–eye coordination and promotes the development of social skills through pretend play and team games.[28]

167

- **Promoting problem solving.** From a young child figuring out how to navigate the monkey bars to older students strategizing during team games and sports, active play offers a wealth of opportunities to practice problem solving. And it provides a key strategy to share with students: Whenever you're stuck on a difficult problem, take a break and go for a run or walk to free the mind for a while. That's when "Eureka!" moments happen!

Reward Your Body with Adequate Rest

Thus far, we've focused on the importance of regular activity for your physical well-being, but adequate sleep is also crucial for a healthy body and brain. In a sleep study involving 147 people ages 20–84, University of Oxford researchers found that lack of sleep caused by difficulty getting to sleep and waking during the night or too early in the morning were linked to a greater-than-average decline in brain volume, particularly in people over the age of 60.[29] More research may be needed to determine whether the reduction in brain volume is a cause or an effect of lack of sleep. Another study of students' sleep habits showed an all-night study session to cram for finals is actually counterproductive, impairing both short-term memory and attention to learning.[30]

Guidelines for healthy sleep for the body and brain suggest that newborns need 16 to 18 hours per day on average, preschoolers need 11 to 12 hours, school-aged children should get at least 10 hours, and teens need 9 to 10 hours. Adults, including the elderly, should aim for 7 to 8 hours of sleep per day.[31] The National Sleep Foundation offers these tips for people who have a hard time getting the sleep they need:

- Maintain a regular sleep and wake schedule, even on the weekends.
- Come up with a regular, relaxing routine in the hour leading up to bedtime. You might try soaking in a warm bath or listening to calming music.

- Make sure your mattress and pillows are comfortable, and keep your bedroom dark, quiet, comfortable, and cool.
- Avoid "sleep stealers," such as reading, watching TV, or using a computer in bed.
- Exercise regularly.
- Finish eating at least two to three hours before bedtime.
- Avoid caffeine and alcohol close to bedtime. Nicotine is a stimulant so giving up smoking will also help avoid sleep problems.[32]

Find What You Love

When you picked up this book, you probably had some personal goals in mind. Those goals might focus on fitness, or they might seem more cerebral. However, research that supports the interrelated nature of the Body–Brain System makes it clear that a commitment to enhancing physical health pays dividends in improved cognitive functioning as well. Even for the brainiest of endeavors, regular physical activity plays an important supporting role.

To accomplish your aim to become positively smarter, fitness should become part of your routine, so it's important to find a form of exercise you enjoy. Some people look forward to a daily walk or run on their own; they appreciate the solitude and the opportunity to either think through perplexing problems or just let their mind wander. Others enjoy more social workouts, such as exercise groups at a fitness center. Still others opt for competitive regimens such as tennis or racquetball. Parents can take advantage of the chance to run, jump, and play while simultaneously modeling the importance of regular exercise as they join their young children on the playground. In his book *Spark: The Revolutionary New Science of Exercise and the Brain*, Harvard professor and physician John Ratey recommends taking up a regular activity such as a dance class or tae kwan do that provides the dual benefits of an aerobic workout and improvements in coordination as a way to boost both body and brain functioning.[33]

169

Making Exercise Part of Your Routine

There are a wide variety of activities you can incorporate in your daily life to bolster your body and brain power, but how much is enough to optimize the impact of aerobic exercise and strength training? The Centers for Disease Control and Prevention offer these guidelines, based on the *2008 Physical Activity Guidelines*.[34]

For kids The activity guidelines call for 60 minutes or more of active play daily for children and adolescents, a theme that has garnered a lot of support from health and sports organizations, including the Heart and Stroke Foundation and the Play 60 Challenge cosponsored by the National Football League and American Heart Association.[35] Their daily play should include aerobic, strength-building, and bone-strengthening activities:

- Aerobic activity of moderate intensity, such as running, riding bikes, jumping rope, playing basketball, or brisk walking, should make up most of kids' 60 minutes.
- Gymnastics, pushups, and other forms of strength training help build strong muscles and healthy bodies.
- Activities like running and jumping rope also support healthy bone development.

For adults The activity guidelines recommend at least 150 minutes (or $2\frac{1}{2}$ hours) of aerobic activity per week and muscle-strengthening activities at least twice a week that work out all major muscle groups (legs, hips, back, abdomen, chest, shoulders, and arms). Even short bursts of 10 minutes or more of moderate or vigorous effort, like running or working out, can have positive health effects. Keep these tips in mind when planning how best to incorporate physical activity into your daily routine:

- Exercise is "aerobic" if it gets you breathing harder and your heart beating faster. A good gauge of engaging in moderate-intensity activity, such as walking fast, doing water aerobics, or riding a bike on a fairly level path, is that you'll be able to talk but not sing. In comparison, engaging in vigorous-intensity activity, such as running, swimming laps, or riding a bike on a hilly trail, means that you won't be able to say more than a few words without pausing for breath.

- To gain the health benefits of muscle-strengthening exercises like lifting weights or doing pushups, you need to keep repeating the activity until it's hard for you to continue without help. A *repetition* is one complete movement of an activity, and a *set* refers to completing several repetitions at one time. For example, you might aim to do 8 to 12 repetitions in one set when you're just beginning a strength-training regimen. Over time you should aim to increase your activity to two or three sets. Yoga, lifting weights, working with resistance bands or equipment, exercises like pushups that use your body weight for resistance, and chores that involve heavy lifting, digging, or shoveling are examples of muscle-strengthening activities.

For older adults If you're 65 or older, generally fit, and have no limiting health conditions, "regular physical activity is one of the most important things you can do for your health," the CDC notes. "It can prevent many of the health problems that seem to come with age. It also helps your muscles grow stronger so you can keep doing your day-to-day activities without becoming dependent on others."[36] The activity guidelines recommend the same amounts of aerobic and muscle-strengthening activities as for younger adults and suggest that upping the ante to 300 minutes (5 hours) per week will produce even greater health benefits.

Putting the Research on Exercise into Personal Practice

Over the years in live events, audiences almost always ask Marcus what he does to put these suggestions into practice. Fair question! Marcus shares the fact that discovering the research set out in Evans and Rosenberg's *Biomarkers* about the importance of strength training for middle-aged and older adults was a revelation that had great personal impact for him and Donna: Before reading that book, I was caught up in the current of conventional wisdom and focused on aerobic exercise, mostly walking along the beach near our home and rowing in the summers back in Cambridge, England. For a spell both Donna and I did some light weight training at the YMCA, which felt good but we were not making much progress. Overall, then, we had a mostly aerobic approach to fitness.

After getting into this research and learning, to my horror, that I could be losing 12 pounds of muscle every 20 years and getting weaker and less vital, I sought out an excellent trainer, Bruce Day, at our local fitness center and invested in regular coaching in how to get optimal results from weight training safely. I was so enthusiastic that I would run to the fitness center and burst through the door ready to work out. I would complete the workout and feel strong and focused for the day. Over just a few months I made great progress. I doubled or tripled my strength on all the exercises and added at least 10 pounds of muscle. In effect I won back about 20 years of muscle loss, and today I feel stronger than ever. While I keep getting occasional support from Bruce on form, I now do my weight training by myself on the road and in the fitness center using what Evans and Couzens in their book *AstroFit* call "E-Centric weight training."[37] Using this approach, you lift the weight on a count of two seconds and lower the weight at the count of six. Evans's research for NASA found that this is optimal for building muscle and strength.

Over the past five years, it has become my routine to engage in weight training on average at least twice a week and most days when we are not traveling. I've developed and maintained a steady regimen without injury and with a high level of enjoyment. Now with the new understandings about the benefits to brain health, Donna and I enjoy boosting our positive outlook and building our brains by lifting weights three or four times a week. It is very motivating.

Low Heart Rate Route to Runners' High

In addition to weight training, I have steadily built up my capacity for running. When I started, I was huffing and puffing over a half-mile. Now I look forward to finishing half-marathons. The key for me has been to adopt a natural running style that focuses on landing lightly on the mid-foot rather than my previous heavy heel-striking style and training at a low heart rate of 180 minus age, as recommended by Philip Maffetone.[38] I usually run every other day and cross-train by cycling, using a rowing machine, or walking to maintain fitness while allowing the legs and feet to recover. The focus is on smart, steady progress. There is not room in this book to go deeper into this approach, but I recommend the website www.naturalrunning.org if you're interested in more information.

Winning Our Blades: A Positive Payoff

I began rowing in "eights" some 40 years ago in my hometown of Cambridge, England. Each year the city hosts a unique event called the Cambridge Town Bumps. This competition takes advantage of the River Cam's narrowness: Crews line up behind each other with the goal of "bumping" the crew in front before being bumped by the crew behind. As has become a summer tradition, I returned to Cambridge in 2014 to row with my crew, many of whom I have rowed with for decades. (These days we row in a lower division, of course.) This summer, after bumping a crew in front on each of the four nights of the competition, we were adorned with strands of victory willow on our row back to the boathouse. We had won our blades! More importantly, we agreed that this was some of our best rowing in recent years. I felt that my running and strength training had helped me to get the most out of this experience and to be better able to keep up with the rest of the crew. Although the decades have progressed, my enjoyment of rowing is as strong as ever. In essence, I have found forms of exercise I enjoy and incorporated them into my routine, as per the recommendations in this chapter. We will be sharing more and updated information about the benefits of different forms of exercise and on topics such as interval training and stretching on www.InnovatingMinds.org.

Notes

1   John J. Ratey and Richard Manning. 2014. *Go Wild: Free Your Body and Mind from the Afflictions of Civilization* (Kindle ed.). New York: Little, Brown, p. 103.

2   Majid Fotuhi. 2013. *Boost Your Brain: The New Art and Science Behind Enhanced Brain Performance.* New York: HarperOne, p. 30.

3   William J. Evans and Irwin H. Rosenberg. 1991. *Biomarkers: The 10 Determinants of Aging You Can Control.* New York: Simon & Schuster, p. 15.

4   Donna Wilson and Marcus Conyers. 2013. *Five Big Ideas for Effective Teaching: Connecting Mind, Brain, and Education Research to Classroom Practice.* New York: Teachers College Press, p. 93.

5   Centers for Disease Control and Prevention. "Press Release: One in Five Adults Meet Overall Physical Activity Guidelines," May 2, 2013. Retrieved from http://www.cdc.gov/media/releases/2013/p0502-physical-activity.html

6   Research America. "Press Release: Top Concerns About Aging: Failing Health, Mental Ability," February 2, 2006. Retrieved from http://www.researchamerica.org/release_06feb2_agingpoll_parade

7   Society for Neuroscience. "Physical Exercise Beefs Up the Brain," August 28, 2013. Retrieved from http://www.brainfacts.org/across-the-lifespan/diet-and-exercise/articles/2013/physical-exercise-beefs-up-the-brain/; Fotuhi, p. 19.

8   S. J. Colcombe, A. F. Kramer, K. I. Erickson, P. Scalf, and colleagues. "Cardiovascular Fitness, Cortical Plasticity, and Aging." *Proceedings of the National Academy of Sciences USA, 101*(9), March 2, 2004, 3316–3321.

9   K. I. Erickson, M. W. Voss, R. S. Prakash, C. Basak, and colleagues. "Exercise Training Increases Size of Hippocampus and Improves Memory." *Proceedings of the National Academy of Sciences USA, 108*(7), February 15, 2011, 3017–3022. Retrieved from http://www.ncbi.nlm.nih.gov/pmc/articles/PMC3041121/

10 S. B. Chapman, S. Aslan, J. S. Spence, L. F. Defina, and colleagues. "Shorter Term Aerobic Exercise Improves Brain, Cognition, and Cardiovascular Fitness in Aging." *Frontiers in Aging Neuroscience, 5,* November 12, 2013. Retrieved from http://www.ncbi.nlm.nih.gov/pmc/articles/PMC3825180/

11 David Hecht. "The Neural Basis of Optimism and Pessimism." *Experimental Neurobiology, 22*(3), September 2013, 173–199. doi: 10.5607/en.2013.22.3.173

12 M. C. Miller. 2011. *Understanding Depression*. Boston: Harvard Medical School.

13 Sharon Begley. "Buff Your Brain: Want to Be Smarter in Work, Love, and Life?" *Newsweek*, January 9 and 16, 2012, p. 33.

14 Christopher Bergland. "Irisin: The 'Exercise Hormone' Has Powerful Health Benefits." The Athlete's Way (blog), February 19, 2014. Retrieved from http://www.psychologytoday.com/blog/the-athletes-way/201402/irisin-the-exercise-hormone-has-powerful-health-benefits; Heidi Godman. "Natural 'Exercise' Hormone Transforms Fat Cells." Harvard Health Blog, June 5, 2012. Retrieved from http://www.health.harvard.edu/blog/natural-exercise-hormone-transforms-fat-cells-201206054851

15 Karl Knopf. 2006. *Weights for 50+: Building Strength, Staying Healthy and Enjoying an Active Lifestyle*. Berkeley, CA: Ulysses Press, p. 11.

16 Evans and Rosenberg, p. 44.

17 Robert Arnot. 1995. *Dr. Bob Arnot's Guide to Turning Back the Clock*. New York: Little, Brown, p. 303.

18 Knopf, p. 8.

19 William J. Evans. "Protein Nutrition, Exercise, and Aging." *Journal of the American College of Nutrition, 23*(6), 2004, 601S–609S.

20 Evans and Rosenberg, pp. 51–52.

21 University of British Columbia. "Physical Activity Can Slow Cognitive Decline, Says UBC Physical Therapist," February 6, 2014. Retrieved from http://news.ubc.ca/2014/02/06/how-exercise-can-boost-brain-power/

22 M. A. I. Aberg, N. I. Pedersen, K. Torén, M. Svartengren, and colleagues. "Cardiovascular Fitness Is Associated with Cognition in Young Adulthood." *Proceedings of the National Academy of Sciences*, 106(49), 2009, 20906–20911. doi: 10.1073/pnas.0905307106

23 James B. Grissom. "Physical Fitness and Academic Achievement." *Journal of Exercise Physiology, 8*(1), 2005, 11–25. Retrieved from http://www.asep.org/files/Grissom.pdf

24 Michele Tine. "Acute Aerobic Exercise: An Intervention for the Selective Visual Attention and Reading Comprehension of Low-Income Adolescents." *Frontiers in Psychology*, June 11, 2014. Retrieved from http://journal.frontiersin.org/Journal/10.3389/fpsyg.2014.00575/full

25 National Center for Chronic Disease Prevention and Health Promotion. 2014. *Health and Academic Achievement*. Atlanta, GA: Centers for Disease Control and Prevention, p. 3. Retrieved from http://www.cdc.gov/healthyyouth/health_and_academics/pdf/health-academic-achievement.pdf

26 Mona Iskander. "A Physical Education in Naperville." *Need to Know on PBS*, February 8, 2011. Retrieved from http://www.pbs.org/wnet/need-to-know/video/a-physical-education-in-naperville-ill/7134/

27 Edward M. Hallowell. 2011. *Shine: Using Brain Science to Get the Best from Your People*. Boston: Harvard Business Review Press, p. 132.

28 Donna Wilson and Marcus Conyers. 2013. *Flourishing in the First Five Years: Connecting Implications from Mind, Brain, and Education Research to the Development of Young Children*. Lanham, MD: Rowman & Littlefield Education, pp. 39–40.

29 Claire E. Sexton, Andreas B. Storsve, Kristine B. Walhovd, Heidi Johansen-Berg, and Anders M. Fjell. "Poor Sleep Quality Is Associated with Increased Cortical Atrophy in Community-Dwelling Adults." *Neurology*, September 3, 2014. doi: 10.1212/WNL.0000000000000774

30 Y. Anwar. "An Afternoon Nap Markedly Boosts the Brain's Learning Capacity," February 22, 2010. Retrieved from http://newscenter.berkeley. edu/2010/02/22/naps_boost_learning_capacity/

31 Centers for Disease Control and Prevention. "How Much Sleep Do I Need?" July 1, 2013. Retrieved from http://www.cdc.gov/sleep/about_ sleep/how_much_sleep.htm

32 National Sleep Foundation. "How Much Sleep Do We Really Need?" Retrieved from http://sleepfoundation.org/how-sleep-works/how-much-sleep-do-we-really-need

33 John J. Ratey. 2008. *Spark: The Revolutionary New Science of Exercise and the Brain*. New York: Little, Brown.

34 Centers for Disease Control and Prevention. "How Much Physical Activity Do You Need?" Retrieved from http://www.cdc.gov/physical-activity/everyone/guidelines/index.html

35 American Heart Association. "Play 60 Challenge" (resources for families and teachers). Retrieved from http://www.heart.org/HEARTORG/ Educator/FortheClassroom/NFLPlay60Challenge/PLAY-60-Challenge-Teacher-Guide_UCM_304758_Article.jsp

36 Centers for Disease Control and Prevention. "How Much Physical Activity Do Older Adults Need? Physical Activity Is Essential to Healthy Aging." Retrieved from http://www.cdc.gov/physicalactivity/ everyone/guidelines/olderadults.html

37 William J. Evans and Gerald Couzens. 2003. *AstroFit: The Astronaut Program for Anti-Aging*. New York: Free Press.

38 Philip Maffetone. 2010. *The Big Book of Endurance Training and Racing*. New York: Skyhorse Publishing, p. 79.

8

Fuel Your Body–Brain System for Peak Performance

"What most people don't know is that the food you eat literally reshapes your brain."

—Majid Fotuhi[1]

In addition to engaging in regular exercise, eating smarter can have a profoundly positive impact on our physical well-being, stoke the achievement of our goals, and support ongoing happiness. The connection between good nutrition and a healthy body is obvious, but emerging science shows that increasing our intake of certain nutrients and avoiding food choices that are high in sugar, saturated fat, and sodium can also boost brain power. By guiding children to develop nutritious eating habits, parents and teachers can help improve their focus on learning and academic achievement and set them on a trajectory to optimize their well-being across the life span. Maintaining those habits into adulthood and later years can support both cardiovascular and brain health. In an article on "Food as Brain Medicine," Fernando Gómez-Pinilla, professor of neurosurgery and physiological science at UCLA, makes the case that:

> Food is like a pharmaceutical compound that affects the brain. Diet, exercise, and sleep have the potential to alter our brain health and mental function. This raises the exciting possibility that changes in diet are a viable strategy for enhancing cognitive abilities, protecting the brain from damage, and counteracting the effects of aging.[2]

Ongoing research offers tantalizing evidence on the protective impact of foods rich in vitamins, omega-3 fatty acids, and other important nutrients to provide high-octane fuel for the Body–Brain System.

Complete the action assessment in Table 8.1 to establish your "baseline" for healthy eating.

Table 8.1 Action Assessment: Choosing Healthy Foods

In your daily diet, do you …	*Almost never*	*Sometimes*	*Frequently*	*Consistently*
1. Make fruits and vegetables part of meals and snacks (nine servings a day, excluding potatoes).				
2. Choose lean protein.				
3. Understand the role of omega-3 fatty acids in maintaining heart and brain health and incorporate these good fats into your diet.				
4. Choose whole grains over refined flours.				

(continued)

Table 8.1   Action Assessment: Choosing Healthy Foods (*cont'd*)

In your daily diet, do you ...	Almost never	Sometimes	Frequently	Consistently
5. Minimize your intake of trans fats, saturated fats, sugar, and sodium.				
6. Pay attention to portion size.				
7. Set positive goals for healthy eating.				

The Brain Benefits of "Going Mediterranean"

A key finding in recent research is that there is no "silver bullet" for healthy eating, no exceptional ingredient that leads the nutritional pack in supporting body and brain functions. Rather, suggest the researchers who studied the connection between eating habits and the incidence of Alzheimer's disease among more than 2,000 older adults living in New York City, "an overall dietary pattern is likely to have a greater effect on health than a single nutrient."[3] In this study, the researchers found that the more closely the eating habits of their subjects adhered to food choices associated with the Mediterranean diet, the less likely they were to develop dementia. The *Mediterranean diet*—rich in fruits and vegetables, beans and nuts, whole grains, fish, and olive oil, with only small amounts of red meat and dairy foods—brings together a host of heart- and brain-healthy nutrients. Writing about the science behind the staples of this cuisine, Walter Willett, who chairs the nutrition department of the Harvard School of Public Health, noted that "together with regular physical activity and not smoking, our analyses suggest that over 80% of coronary heart disease, 70% of stroke, and 90% of type 2 diabetes can be avoided by healthy food choices that are consistent with the traditional Mediterranean diet."[4]

On the other side of the country, research as part of the Oregon Brain Aging Study on the impact of dietary choices identified five nutrients that were high in the blood levels of subjects who scored well on tests assessing memory, attention, and language processing: vitamins B, C, D, and E and omega-3 fatty acids.[5] Conversely, people with high levels of trans fats in their diets registered lower on the tests of cognitive performance and had less total cerebral volume than subjects with lower levels of that form of fat, typically found in packaged, fast, fried, and frozen foods, in their blood samples. "These results need to be confirmed, but obviously it is very exciting to think that people could potentially stop their brains from shrinking and keep them sharp by adjusting their diet" to increase their vitamin and omega-3 intake and eliminate trans fats, lead researcher Gene Bowman noted.[6]

In related research, Bowman and his colleagues also found that older adults with higher levels of omega-3 fatty acids in their blood samples exhibited fewer lesions in the white matter of their brains; white matter lesions are associated with dementia and cognitive decline.[7] These subjects also did better on tests of executive function. This research is among the most recent in a growing body of evidence that omega-3s enhance blood flow throughout the body and brain and increase the brain chemical BDNF, which supports neurogenesis and synaptogenesis.[8]

In sum, these findings suggest that the food choices that are good for the heart are also good for the brain. Omega-3 fatty acids are polyunsaturated fats with anti-inflammatory properties that help protect against cardiovascular disease and stroke and may also provide some benefits for people with cancer, asthma, and autoimmune diseases. The body doesn't produce omega-3s, so you need to ensure they are included in the foods you eat. Nutritional supplements are also an option. Look for foods and supplements that include EPA (eicosapentaenoic acid) and DHA (docosahexaenoic acid), which are long-chain omega-3s found in salmon, tuna, sardines, trout, and other seafood; DHA is also found in algae. Another member of this family, ALA (alpha-linolenic acid, a short-chain omega-3), is found in plants such as flaxseed, spinach, broccoli, cauliflower, and some beans and nuts.

What's on Your Plate?

As noted, vitamins and omega-3s are only part of the story when it comes to food choices that nurture the Body–Brain System. The Healthy Eating Plate (see Figure 8.1), developed by nutrition specialists at the Harvard School of Public Health and editors at Harvard Health Publications, provides a simple, easy-to-understand guide to creating healthy, balanced meals:

- A variety of colorful fruits and vegetables should occupy the largest portion of your plate.
- Whole grains like whole wheat, barley, wheat berries, quinoa, oats, and brown rice and the foods made with them have a

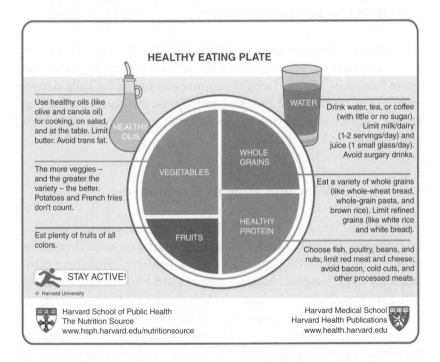

Figure 8.1 The Healthy Eating Plate, recommendations from the Harvard School of Public Health. As printed in image and © Harvard University. For more information visit: www.health.harvard.edu

milder effect on blood sugar than refined grains and support weight management and gastrointestinal health.

- Protein is an essential nutrient necessary for creating and repairing cells and supporting healthy organs, bones, and blood supply. The healthiest sources of protein are fish, chicken, beans, and nuts.
- Healthy vegetable oils include olive, canola, soy, corn, sunflower, and peanut oils. Avoid partially hydrogenated oils, which contain unhealthy trans fats, and remember that a "low-fat" label on oils and margarines does not mean they are healthy, the Harvard nutritionists advise.
- Staying hydrated is crucial. The healthiest drink choices are water, coffee, or tea. Limit milk and dairy intake to one or two servings a day, and limit fruit juice to one small glass daily. Skip soda and sugary drinks altogether.

The final graphic component of the Healthy Eating Plate is the running figure, a reminder to stay active to support body and brain health. With this helpful summary in mind, let's dig deeper into recent research on effective nutritional strategies to support higher cognitive performance, positive mood, enhanced energy, and greater well-being.

Why and How to Eat Smarter

Vitamins are vital to your vitality Thirteen essential vitamins, including vitamins A, C, D, E, and K and eight types of B vitamins such as riboflavin (B2) and folate (B9), perform critical supporting roles in helping our bodies convert food into energy, maintain cells, and support immune systems. Extended deprivation of vitamins can cause serious medical conditions. For example, a deficiency of vitamin B12 can cause anemia and neurological problems such as depression, dementia, and memory loss. As much as possible, you should aim to get the vitamins you need in your daily diet rather than relying on vitamin supplements. While an article from the Harvard School of Public Health suggests that "a daily multivitamin is a great nutrition insurance policy,"[9] one recent study raises questions about the potentially counterproductive effect of taking supplements while engaging in a strenuous fitness regimen. Exercise buffs participating in the study who took a placebo showed more mitochondrial growth (structures in cells that produce energy) than those taking vitamin supplements.[10] In short, vitamin supplements should not replace a healthy diet, but they may be helpful in some cases, especially for pregnant women and people with specific medical conditions or at higher risk for heart disease or cancer.

The antioxidants in fruits and vegetables are good for the brain and body Researchers are finding that these protective properties are especially important for older adults. As the brain ages, nerve cells are less able to protect themselves from the damage done by free radicals through a process known as oxidative stress, which is related to mental decline and other age-related degenerative diseases. Antioxidants in well-known nutrients, including vitamins C and E, beta carotene, and selenium, are all present in abundance in fruits, vegetables, nuts, and whole grains. Research funded by the US Department of Agriculture reveals that these antioxidants not only counter brain decline, but may help head off cancer as well.[11]

Flavonoids help paint a picture of health Flavonoids are plant pigments that give fruits and vegetables their rich colors—and provide humans with a variety of health benefits. In addition to antioxidant and anti-inflammatory properties, some of these compounds have been found to increase BDNF and promote neurogenesis in the hippocampus. Others may improve blood flow and activate mitochondria in cells to enhance their release of energy.[12] Examples of foods rich in flavonoids include beets, blueberries, and cocoa (for more information on these "power foods," see the following section).

Flavonoids are one group of phytochemicals, or compounds in food known to have protective properties. These chemicals are found in colorful fruits and vegetables that are not only gorgeous to look at and delicious to eat but color-coded for your health. A good rule of thumb is that the deeper the color, the better they may be for you.[13] For example:

- The anthocyanins in blueberries, blackberries, cranberries, and purple-colored grains (corn, rice, and potato varieties) may have antimicrobial properties, help to reduce inflammation, and prevent oxidative damage to cells.
- Carotenoids enrich the yellow, orange, and red colors of many fruits and vegetables. These pigments include beta-carotene, which contributes to vision and bone health and supports the immune system (and can be found in carrots, oranges, and cantaloupe); lycopene, which is being studied as a possible cancer preventative (tomatoes); and lutein, which may protect the eyes from the damaging effects of sunlight and reduce the risk of macular degeneration (spinach, kale, and turnip greens).
- Chlorophylls found in green leafy vegetables are also rich in lutein and may work with another food chemical, zeaxanthin (found in peppers and grapes), to help protect the eyes.

Out with the bad fats, in with the good The medical evidence against trans fats, which are found in margarine and vegetable shortening and thus in baked and fried foods using them as ingredients, has finally begun to steamroll these hydrogenated fats out of American diets. Recent research presented to the American Heart Association finds that trans fats not only have a negative impact on the cardiovascular system but also impair brain functioning and memory.[14] With recent FDA requirements aiming to phase out trans fats and state and local regulations outlawing the use of these ingredients, many fast-food restaurants have discontinued their use, and many snack products now bear the label "No trans fats." That doesn't mean those products are healthy, though; they may still be made with saturated fats, which are also known to increase overall cholesterol, especially LDL (or "bad cholesterol"). Saturated fats are found in meat and dairy products, cocoa butter, and coconut oil. Foods high in saturated fats and sugar may play a role in reduced cognitive functioning and memory loss as we age.[15]

On the other hand, monounsaturated and polyunsaturated fats have been found to have positive effects on blood cholesterol levels by reducing LDL and increasing HDL (a.k.a., "good cholesterol"). Monounsaturated fats are found in seeds, nuts, olive oil, and avocados, while salmon, albacore tuna, mackerel, and sardines are good sources of polyunsaturated fats. These nutrients are good for the brain as well. In particular, as we have noted previously, the omega-3 fatty acids found in fish oils are powerful nutrients that may help transmit signals between brain cells.

All in for whole grains   In 2010, researchers for the American Society for Nutrition enumerated a wealth of findings that adding whole grains to your diet can lower the risk of chronic diseases, including coronary heart disease, diabetes, and cancer, and contribute to weight management and gastrointestinal health.[16] Researchers continue to study what components of whole grains— the fiber, vitamins, minerals, antioxidants, phenolic acids, and/or phytochemicals—offer this protective effect.

At any rate, the USDA's 2010 *Dietary Guidelines for Americans* recommend that at least half of all grains you eat are whole grains, which leads to the question: What exactly are whole grains? They are unrefined grains with bran and germ intact which makes them better sources of fiber and other nutrients than refined grains with the brain and germ removed. Examples of whole-grain foods include brown rice, popcorn, whole wheat bread, and buckwheat pancakes.

Forget sugar highs. Protein has staying power   Unlike sugary treats that produce a short-term "sugar high" followed quickly by a crash that leaves you feeling sleepy and without energy, a meal featuring lean protein can help fuel laser-sharp attention. According to research from the Reynolds Center on Aging, a healthy diet with adequate sources of lean protein can also help reverse age-related muscle loss.[17] Excellent sources of lean protein include fish (which, depending on the type of fish, may also supply omega-3 fatty acids), white-meat poultry (remove the skin before you cook it), low-fat dairy products, eggs, beans, and soy.

185

Watch your portions With all the talk about good fats vs. bad fats and whole grains vs. refined grains, the reality is that an occasional decadent treat won't ruin your health. In fact, many foods can be part of a healthy eating habit as long as they are consumed in moderation. Eggs are a good example. They add protein to your daily intake and may also be an important source of lutein, but like other animal proteins, egg yolks contain saturated fats. That's why the USDA Food Pyramid lists one or two eggs as a healthy single portion. Here are some other portion guidelines from the food pyramid:

- Protein: 2–3 ounces of meat (about the size of a deck of cards or the palm of your hand); two tablespoons of almond or peanut butter; one-third cup of dry beans.
- Grains: One slice of whole grain bread; 1 ounce of prepared cereal; one-half cup of pasta or rice.
- Fruits or vegetables: one apple, orange, or banana, for example; one-half cup of chopped fruit or vegetable; three-fourths cup of fruit juice.
- Dairy products: one cup of milk; $1\frac{1}{2}$ ounces of cheese (look for low-fat or fat-free options).

Reduce sodium intake According to the American Heart Association, 9 out of 10 people consume much more than the recommended amounts of sodium, which is associated with high blood pressure. The recommended daily dose is 1,500 milligrams; Americans consume on average 3,400 milligrams. Most of the excess salt in our diets comes in prepared foods purchased at supermarkets and convenience stores (65 percent) and restaurants (25 percent). Lose the salt shaker, check the sodium content on food labels, and choose low sodium alternatives.[18]

Apply your positive outlook to healthy eating In keeping with our view of the power of an optimistic perspective, Susan Raatz, writing for the Agricultural Research Service, shares findings that a negative approach to nutritional advice—"Don't eat sweets," "Avoid fats," etc.—has proven largely unsuccessful. Instead, she suggests that focusing on what and how you should eat will likely produce more progress toward making healthy eating habits a way of life.[19] Toward that end, Raatz offers these recommendations:

1. Balance daily calorie intake by finding out how many calories you need (Raatz recommends www.ChooseMyPlate.gov as a good starting point) and finding opportunities every day to be physically active.
2. Enjoy what you eat by eating more slowly and paying attention to your food choices instead of being distracted by reading or watching TV during meal time. When you take your time, you're more likely to notice signs that you are getting full, so you'll eat less as well.
3. Use a smaller plate, bowl, and glass, and measure your portions. When eating out, choose a smaller size portion, share a dish, or ask for a bag to take part of your meal home.
4. Eat more vegetables, fruits, whole grains, and low-fat dairy products for meals and snacks.
5. Make half your plate vegetables and substitute fruit for sugary, fatty desserts. And remember, the more colorful, the better.
6. Make at least half your grains whole. Eat whole wheat bread and muffins instead of baked goods made with refined flour and brown rice instead of white rice.
7. Compare sodium content in canned and frozen foods. Opt for foods labeled "low sodium," "reduced sodium," and "no salt added."
8. Drink plenty of water instead of sugary drinks. Soda, energy drinks, and sports drinks are a major source of added sugar and calories in American diets.

Substituting flavorful fresh fruits and vegetables, whole grains, and lean protein for sugary, salt-laden prepared foods offers a delicious, healthy menu. You don't need to feel like you're being deprived. Instead treat your Body–Brain System to choices that are good to eat and good for you!

Better by the Dozen: Twelve Power Foods to Fuel Well-Being

There's a lot of talk these days about "powerhouse foods," especially fruits and vegetables associated with improving health and warding off disease. But there is no accepted standard for classifying these foods, so dietary researcher Jennifer Di Noia set out to offer one, applying the title *powerhouse* to foods that supply 10 percent or more daily value of 17 qualifying nutrients (potassium, fiber, protein, calcium, iron, thiamin, riboflavin, niacin, folate, zinc, and vitamins A, B6, B12, C, D, E, and K) for each 100 kilocalories per 100 grams of the fruit or vegetable.[20]

After proposing those parameters, Di Noia then tested 47 foods touted for their health benefits against this standard and ranked the 41 that qualified as sufficiently nutrient dense. Watercress topped the list, followed by other leafy green vegetables: Chinese cabbage, chard, beet greens, spinach, chicory, leaf lettuce, parsley, romaine lettuce, and collard, turnip, and mustard greens. Farther down the list, but still making the cut were cabbage, carrots, tomatoes, lemons, strawberries, radishes, winter squash, oranges, limes, grapefruit, rutabaga, turnips, blackberries, leeks, and sweet potatoes.

In addition to this list, at least a dozen other foods are worthy of consideration as "power foods," based on the research for their health benefits.

1. **Blueberries.** Tufts University researchers suggest that of all the major organs studied, the brain has the lowest level of antioxidant capacity.[21] This means that the brain may be particularly vulnerable to free radical damage. Researchers have found that blueberries are among the most potent sources of antioxidants. In one experiment, rats fed a blueberry-infused diet demonstrated better spatial memory and quicker learning than rats who ate a control diet, and higher levels of BDNF were found in their hippocampi.[22]

2. **Nuts.** Harvard nutritional expert Walter Willett reports that people who regularly eat nuts have a 30 to 50 percent lower

risk of heart attack or heart disease, based on a review of major cohort studies.[23] Fotuhi suggests that pecans and pistachios are a good source of the nutrient choline, which may increase production of the memory-related neurotransmitter acetylcholine.[24]

3. **Salmon.** In addition to the benefits cited previously, research by University of Chicago professor Michael Roizen indicates that eating fish rich in omega-3 fatty acids once a week can halve the risk of heart attack.[25]

4. **Spinach.** No. 5 on Di Noia's list of powerhouse vegetables is singled out here for its prominence in other nutrition research. Animal studies at Tufts University indicate that spinach is excellent in maintaining brain function and slowing the aging process. Low levels of folic acid in the diet may help maintain high levels of the amino acid homocysteine in the blood, which may contribute to cardiovascular disease.[26] The daily recommended intake of folic acid is 400 micrograms; a cup of cooked spinach delivers 262 mcg of folic acid, which would put you well on your way to meeting this nutritional goal!

5. **Frozen yogurt.** This popular treat is a healthy and delicious substitute for ice cream. Research suggests that yogurt can be a good source of calcium, with 400 mg per serving.

6. **Olive oil.** The Food and Drug Administration's decision to phase out trans fats ultimately could save 7,000 Americans from premature death and prevent three times as many nonfatal heart attacks.[27] Switching to heart-healthy substitutes such as olive oil can reduce those risks and add extra flavor to your favorite dishes.

7. **Brown bread.** The American Society for Nutrition's findings about the many benefits of whole grains supports recommendations to avoid the insulin rush that may be caused by white flour products such as donuts, bagels, and white bread. Instead, switch to whole wheat bread, which is higher in fiber and causes less of a spike in insulin levels.

8. **Tomatoes.** David Snowdon of the Sanders-Brown Aging Center at the University of Kentucky is director of the

well-known "nun study" on aging. Among other findings, his research noted that study participants with the lowest levels of lycopene in their blood had the highest levels of cognitive decline and were four times more likely to need assisted living than those with higher levels of this protective nutrient.[28] Animal studies have found that lycopene may have a cancer-preventative effect, although research with humans has produced inconclusive results.[29] Tomatoes are a prime source of lycopene, which seems to be best absorbed when they are cooked and consumed with a little fat.

9. **Green tea.** According to the Agricultural Research Service, green tea is an excellent example of the power of phytonutrients, the plant-based compounds that provide a wide range of health benefits. Chief among these protections are antioxidative and anti-inflammatory properties that have been shown to counteract oxidative stress and inflammation in the arteries, reducing the risk of developing atherosclerosis. Green tea contains high amounts of epigallocatecin gallate (EGCG), a powerful natural antioxidant.[30]

10. **Bananas.** Roizen's research has also established that increasing consumption of potassium may reduce the risk of stroke. One study showed people who ate low levels of potassium had a 2.6 to 4.8 times higher risk of stroke than people who regularly consumed bananas and other fruits and vegetables rich in potassium.

11. **Turmeric.** This spice and its active ingredient, curcumin, are being studied for their possible health benefits.[31] Fotuhi cites research that curcumin acts as an anti-inflammatory and increases blood flow to the brain and suggests that the much lower incidence of Alzheimer's disease in India (about one-quarter that of the United States), where curcumin is a staple in the diet, may provide possible evidence of its brain-protective effects.[32]

12. **Chocolate.** And now for a sweet treat to finish off our power-foods list. That's right, chocolate. The dark kind of chocolate (with at least 70 percent cocoa content) is rich in flavonoids, another class of antioxidants that some research links to

190

brain health. Researchers with the Harvard Medical School reported on a study indicating that eating a small amount of dark chocolate may help stave off heart failure and reduce blood pressure.[33] The study of Swedish women found that eating one to three servings of high-quality chocolate, with higher cocoa content and lower sugar, per month was associated with a reduced risk of heart failure. The researchers pinpointed servings of about one-half to two-thirds the size of a typical American chocolate bar and cautioned that the benefits disappeared and even reversed with more frequent chocolate treats (twice a week or more often).

As research continues to explore the role of diet in body and brain health, we certainly have enough evidence to champion choosing foods rich in vitamins, omega-3 fatty acids, and other nutrients with antioxidant and anti-inflammatory properties and low in sugar and saturated fats. Combined with regular aerobic activity and strength training, enjoying healthy foods supports your mental and physical well-being.

Educational Implications of Becoming "HealthWise"

Research is also ongoing to investigate the impact of healthy nutrition, or the lack thereof, on school performance. One recent literature survey cautions that, for the developing minds of children and adolescents, "it can be as dangerous to have too much 'bad' food, as it is to have too little 'good' food ... in helping the brain best capitalize on cognitive capabilities."[34] Food insufficiency—especially an inadequate intake of essential nutrients such as vitamins A, B6, B12, C, and folate and iron, zinc, and calcium—is associated with lower academic performance, higher rates of absenteeism, and an inability to focus on learning, according to a report from the Centers for Disease Control and Prevention. School breakfast and lunch programs provide a much-needed health and learning boost for students from low-income families, the study concludes: "Student participation in the USDA School Breakfast Program is associated with increased academic grades and standardized test scores, reduced absenteeism, and improved cognitive performance."[35] In short, "healthy students are better learners," and ensuring that all children and adolescents have access to an adequate supply of nutritious foods and education about the importance of healthy food choices should be a crucial mission of families, schools, and communities.

Along the same lines, a Canadian study of more than 5,000 fifth graders in Nova Scotia concluded that students with a healthy diet, characterized as including plenty of fruits, vegetables, and whole grains and relatively little fat and sugar, performed better academically than students with a poor diet. These findings led the researchers to call for "investment in effective school nutrition programs that have the potential to improve student access to healthy food choices, diet quality, academic performance, and, over the long term, health."[36]

In the early 2000s, we had the privilege of working with students and teachers at Brookshire Elementary School in Winter Park, Florida, in creating the BrainSMART® HealthWise program to teach children about the benefits of healthy eating. This multifaceted program involved sharing research about how smart food choices and regular exercise can improve body and brain functioning. We consulted with school staff, students, and their parents on the most effective ways to incorporate nutritious food choices into meals and snacks at school and at home, and we designed the HealthMath curriculum as an interdisciplinary approach to explore and emphasize the benefits of healthy eating. The program also emphasized simple steps such as making sure that bottled water was readily available so that students stayed well hydrated and less thirsty for sugary drinks.

An independent assessment of the program revealed a "significant improvement" in the number of students who were overweight or at risk of becoming overweight after participating in the BrainSMART HealthWise Project.[37] Winter Park Health Foundation's vice president, Debbie Watson, reports that after learning about the benefits of healthy habits, students who reported more nutritious food choices, adequate hydration, and regular exercise habits performed better academically. School records indicated an overall decrease in absenteeism and evidence of decreased classroom management issues, and teachers and other school staff and students' families were supportive of the emphasis on developing healthy habits. The Winter Park Foundation BrainSMART HealthWise initiative has become a model for Orange County Public School District.[38] We enjoyed our interactions with students, teachers, and parents and the opportunity to see firsthand how learning about taking charge of one's health can have a transformative impact.

Our work in writing for educators and the general public, presenting at conferences and professional development sessions, and developing the graduate degree courses for teachers has been strongly influenced by the research on the impact of healthy food choices and regular exercise on brain and body health. In particular, we have been inspired by the work of Walter Willett and the Harvard School of Public Health in disseminating research and developing the Harvard Healthy Eating Plan. This research-based approach has influenced our work and our personal health habits, and we believe that getting the word out about these findings has the potential to alleviate a major cause of death and disability in the United States and other countries. A key impetus for writing this book is to help educate children and adults about the positive impact of their health decisions to incorporate healthy eating and physical activity into their daily lives with the big picture goal of becoming positively smarter! For more detailed information about healthy eating, we suggest a visit to http://www.hsph.harvard.edu/nutritionsource/.

Notes

1 Majid Fotuhi. 2013. *Boost Your Brain: The New Art and Science Behind Enhanced Brain Performance.* New York: HarperOne, p. 75.
2 Stuart Wolpert and Mark Wheeler. "Food as Brain Medicine." *UCLA Magazine Online*, July 9, 2008. Retrieved from http://magazine.ucla.edu/exclusives/food_brain_medicine/

3   Nikolaos Scarmeas, Yaakov Stern, Ming-Xin Tang, Richard Mayeux, and Jose Luchsinger. "Mediterranean Diet and Risk for Alzheimer's Disease. *Annals of Neurology,* 59(6), June 2006, 912–921. Retrieved from http://www.ncbi.nlm.nih.gov/pmc/articles/PMC3024594/

4   Walter C. Willett. "The Mediterranean Diet: Science and Practice." *Public Health Nutrition,* 9(1A), February 2006, p. 105.

5   G. L. Bowman, L. C. Silbert, D. Howieson, H. H. Dodge, and colleagues. "Nutrient Biomarker Patterns, Cognitive Function, and MRI Measures of Brain Aging." *Neurology,* December 28, 2011 (published online before print). Retrieved from http://www.natap.org/2012/HIV/Neurology-2011-Bowman-WNL.0b013e3182436598.pdf

6   Fisher Center for Alzheimer's Research Foundation. "5 Nutrients May Promote Brain Health." Retrieved from http://www.alzinfo.org/04/articles/prevention-and-wellness/5-nutrients-promote-brain-health

7   Gene L. Bowman, Hiroko H. Dodge, Nora Mattek, Aron K. Barbey, and colleagues. "Plasma Omega-3 PUFA and White Matter Mediated Executive Decline in Older Adults." *Frontiers in Aging Neuroscience,* 5 (article 92), December 2013. Retrieved from http://journal.frontiersin.org/Journal/10.3389/fnagi.2013.00092/abstract

8   Fotuhi, p. 80.

9   Harvard School of Public Health. "The Nutrition Source: Vitamins." Retrieved from http://www.hsph.harvard.edu/nutritionsource/what-should-you-eat/vitamins/

10 Gretchen Reynolds. "Why Vitamins May Be Bad for Your Workout." *The New York Times,* February 12, 2014. Retrieved from http://well.blogs.nytimes.com/2014/02/12/why-vitamins-may-be-bad-for-your-workout/?_php=true&_type=blogs&_r=0

11 US Department of Agriculture. "Nutrition and Brain Function: Food for the Aging Mind." *Agricultural Research,* August 2007. Retrieved from http://www.ars.usda.gov/is/AR/archive/aug07/aging0807.htm

12 Fotuhi, pp. 82–84.

13 Matthew Picklo. "The Healthy Colors of Your Diet," April 28, 2011. Retrieved from the Agricultural Research Service http://www.ars.usda.gov/News/docs.htm?docid=21735

14 Dennis Thompson. "Trans Fats May Sap Your Memory," November 19, 2014. Retrieved from http://www.everydayhealth.com/news/trans-fats-sap-your-memory/

15 Mehmet Oz and Michael Roizen. "Food for Memory: 5 Foods That Age Your Brain," January 16, 2012. Retrieved from http://www.huffington-post.com/2012/01/16/food-for-memory_n_1197790.html

16 S. S. Jonnalagadda, L. Harnack, R. H. Liu, N. McKeown, and colleagues. 2010. "Putting the Whole Grain Puzzle Together: Health Benefits Associated with Whole Grains—Summary of American

Society for Nutrition 2010 Satellite Symposium." Retrieved from http://www.wholegrainscouncil.org/files/ASNsummary2010.pdf

17 William J. Evans and Gerald Couzens. 2003. *AstroFit: The Astronaut Program for Anti-Aging.* New York: Free Press.

18 American Heart Association. "The Effects of Excess Sodium on Your Health and Appearance." Retrieved from http://www.heart.org/HEARTORG/GettingHealthy/NutritionCenter/HealthyDietGoals/The-Effects-of-Excess-Sodium-on-Your-Health-and-Appearance_UCM_454387_Article.jsp

19 Susan Raatz. "Improve Your Diet with a Positive Approach," September 20, 2011. Retrieved from the Agricultural Research Service http://www.ars.usda.gov/News/docs.htm?docid=22092

20 Jennifer Di Noia. "Defining Powerhouse Fruits and Vegetables: A Nutrient Density Approach." *Preventing Chronic Disease, 11,* June 5, 2014. Retrieved from http://www.cdc.gov/pcd/issues/2014/13_0390.htm#table2_down

21 Marjorie Howard. "Finding the Triggers for Parkinson's Disease." *Tufts Journal,* March 3, 2010. Retrieved from http://tuftsjournal.tufts.edu/2010/03_1/features/01/

22 Fotuhi, pp. 83–84.

23 Walter Willett. 2005. *The Harvard Medical School Guide: Eat, Drink, and Be Healthy.* New York: Simon & Schuster.

24 Fotuhi, p. 85.

25 Michael Roizen. 2001. *The Realage Diet: Make Yourself Younger with What You Eat.* New York: HarperCollins.

26 American Heart Association. "Homocysteine, Folic Acid and Cardiovascular Disease," March 18, 2014. Retrieved from http://www.heart.org/HEARTORG/GettingHealthy/NutritionCenter/Homocysteine-Folic-Acid-and-Cardiovascular-Disease_UCM_305997_Article.jsp

27 Melissa Healy. "FDA's Trans Fat Decision: An Opening for Regulating Salt, Sugar?" *The Los Angeles Times,* November 3, 2013. Retrieved from http://articles.latimes.com/2013/nov/08/science/la-sci-fda-transfat-salt-sugar-regulation-20131107

28 David Snowdon. 2002. *Aging with Grace: What the Nun Study Teaches Us About Leading Longer, Healthier, and More Meaningful Lives.* New York: Bantam.

29 National Cancer Institute. "Prostate Cancer, Nutrition, and Dietary Supplements: Lycopene," June 24, 2014. Retrieved from http://www.cancer.gov/cancertopics/pdq/cam/prostatesupplements/healthprofessional/page3

30 Jay Cao. "Phytonutrients Are Good for Bone Health," November 22, 2011. Retrieved from the Agricultural Research Service http://www.ars.usda.gov/News/docs.htm?docid=22242

31 University of Maryland Medical Center. "Turmeric," May 4, 2011. Retrieved from http://umm.edu/health/medical/altmed/herb/turmeric

32 Fotuhi, p. 85.
33 Amanda Gardner. "Small Amounts of Dark Chocolate May Guard Against Heart Failure." *HealthDay*, August 16, 2010. Retrieved from http://consumer.healthday.com/vitamins-and-nutritional-information-27/food-and-nutrition-news-316/small-amounts-of-dark-chocolate-may-guard-against-heart-failure-642179.html
34 Rita Rausch. "Nutrition and Academic Performance in School-Age Children: The Relation to Obesity and Food Insufficiency." *Journal of Nutrition & Food Sciences, 3*(2), 2013. Retrieved from http://omicsonline.org/nutrition-and-academic-performance-in-school-age-children-the-relation%20to-obesity-and-food-insufficiency-2155-9600.1000190.pdf
35 National Center for Chronic Disease Prevention and Health Promotion. 2014. *Health and Academic Achievement.* Atlanta, GA: Centers for Disease Control and Prevention, p. 2. Retrieved from http://www.cdc.gov/healthyyouth/health_and_academics/pdf/health-academic-achievement.pdf
36 M. D. Florence, M. Asbridge, and P. J. Veugelers. "Diet Quality and Academic Performance." *Journal of School Health, 78*(4), April 2008, 209–215. Retrieved from http://onlinelibrary.wiley.com/doi/10.1111/j.1746-1561.2008.00288.x/full
37 S. Wang and N. Ellis. 2005. *Evaluating the BrainSMART/Health Wise/Health School Team Program at Brookshire Elementary School: An Analysis of BMI Trend Data from 2001 to 2004.* Winter Park, FL: Winter Park Health Foundation.
38 Debbie Watson. 2010. "Healthy Kids Make Better Students" [PowerPoint presentation]. Winter Park, FL: Winter Park Health Foundation.

9

Bringing It All Together, Putting It into Practice

"Successfully intelligent people defy negative expectations, even when these expectations arise from low scores on IQ or similar tests. They do not let other people's assessments stop them from achieving their goals. They find their path and then pursue it, realizing that there will be obstacles along the way and that surmounting these obstacles is part of their challenge."

—Robert J. Sternberg[1]

In the process of developing skills for becoming positively smarter, we may have some misconceptions to confront, some new attitudes to adopt, and some habits to replace. Like the example in the Introduction of the Harvard grads explaining with great confidence what causes winter and summer, we need to step back and carefully examine the most fundamental perceptions of our "private universe" about our potential to become happier, to increase achievement, and to enhance our physical well-being. We must first embrace the fact that we have a tremendous capacity to change.

This is no simple matter. The Innate Talent Paradigm is deeply rooted in assumptions and behaviors at the societal level, and the consequences are far-reaching. Assumptions persist that people

Positively Smarter: Science and Strategies for Increasing Happiness, Achievement, and Well-Being, First Edition. Marcus Conyers and Donna Wilson.
© 2015 John Wiley & Sons, Inc. Published 2015 by John Wiley & Sons, Inc.

are either born optimists or born pessimists and that it is impossible to change one's outlook; that enduring happiness is largely due to external events such as getting a promotion or a bigger house, starting a new relationship, or earning a higher income; that a chosen few are genetically endowed with the "gift" of musical, artistic, academic, or athletic ability; that IQ scores are the sole factor that dictate future achievement; that if disadvantaged students begin school behind their peers, they lack the capacity to catch up and learn the higher-order skills they need to thrive in school and in life; that life span and health status are mostly determined by genetic destiny. These perceptions exert a powerful gravitational pull that is hard to break free from, partly because their influence permeates thoughts and actions at an unconscious level.

Marcus sees this dynamic in action at the individual level when presenting at live events: I'll ask for a show of hands of people who lack the talent for art. Often some 90 percent of the audience raise their hands. Then I ask them how old they were when they discovered they couldn't "do" art. The typical range of responses is between age 6 and 9. Some people will share what led to their discovery, perhaps an off-handed comment from a teacher or the realization that their drawings were never chosen for display in class. I often hear a variation of the comment that "my brother was the artist in the family, and I was the athlete"—as if we can only be one or the other, as if because of our childhood interests and less-than-successful first efforts, some doors are closed to us forever.

The same discussion might have played out if I'd asked, "How many of you are naturally good at math?" or "Do you think of yourself as a good presenter?" And yet, the skills at the foundations of these endeavors—creativity, analytical abilities, problem solving, and effective communication—are prized among job candidates in today's global economy. And more to our central point, they can all be learned and improved. If I'd asked, "What do you think your life span will be?" many people might think first about the longevity of their parents and grandparents—even though genes account for only 25 to 30 percent of our health status and outlook for longevity and our behaviors are much more indicative of long-term health outcomes.

The price we pay as a society for these deeply held, but often unacknowledged, misperceptions is immense, accounted for in lost opportunities. On a personal level, we may avoid investing our time and energy into developing new skills and applying strategies that can change our lives by helping us to become happier and healthier and achieve whatever goals we set for ourselves.

Forging a New Foundation Grounded in Neuroplasticity

The Untapped Potential Paradigm offers a worldview through the lens of the brain's tremendous capacity to change as a result of learning. It provides a more nuanced view of what is possible. When we apply this view in our everyday lives, we come to realize that our intellect and abilities are malleable and can be improved through conscious effort over time. We understand that we can adopt a more optimistic outlook and in doing so achieve greater happiness and more positive relationships with others. And we accept that we can take control of our well-being and improve our body and brain health.

The CIA strategy is a useful tool in establishing this paradigm as our foundation for accepting and accomplishing new challenges:

- We take **control** of how we think, what we know, and what we can do—and work to change our attitudes, knowledge, and skills when necessary.
- We hone in on what **influences** our thoughts and actions, including the possibility that deep-seated misconceptions might be steering us in the wrong direction.
- We **acknowledge** that some changes may require hard work and determination over the long term.

Some changes, though, aren't all that difficult. They just require that we be willing to take control—and take action. In Dan

Millman's semi-autobiographical *Way of the Peaceful Warrior,* a character tells a humorous story about Sam:

> "I met him on a construction site in the Midwest. When the lunch whistle blew, all the workers would sit down together to eat. And every day, Sam would open his lunch pail and start to complain.
>
> "'Son of a gun!' he'd cry, 'not peanut butter and jelly sandwiches again. I hate peanut butter and jelly!'
>
> "He whined about his peanut butter and jelly sandwiches day after day, until one of the guys on the work crew finally said, 'Fer crissakes, Sam, if you hate peanut butter and jelly so much, why don't you just tell yer ol' lady to make you something different?'
>
> "'What do you mean my ol' lady?' Sam replied. 'I'm not married. I make my own sandwiches.'"[2]

By staying stuck in the Innate Talent Paradigm, each of us may be putting up with our own version of peanut butter and jelly sandwiches. But if we adopt the Untapped Potential Paradigm as our foundation, we can set aside the limiting misconceptions about the influence of inborn traits for domains such as art, creativity, math, science, public speaking, greater levels of happiness, achievement, and health and longevity. Imagine how this new outlook would increase inspiration and motivation. The emerging science we have shared in this book is truly inspiring in terms of gathering evidence for the neurocognitive and physical potential to become good, better, and even excellent in almost any domain.

People who set challenging goals for themselves and then develop and follow a plan to attain those goals are often surprised when they achieve, and even surpass, their aims. History books, newscasts, and entertainment media are filled with profiles of successful people who have made the most of their talents and worked hard to achieve their full potential. The only limitation of these success stories is that they tend to showcase their subjects as "extraordinary," when in reality all of us have tremendous potential to learn new skills and accomplish our goals to become positively smarter.

Examples of the UP Paradigm in Practice

Fortunately, there are many examples of the Untapped Potential Paradigm thriving all around us. Workplace studies show that all employees benefit when they receive training on using cognitive strategies to work smarter, with the biggest gains in work performance—up to 400 percent—among women and minorities.[3] In a hypercompetitive global economy, businesses can no longer rely on a "talented few"; supporting the majority of the workforce to improve their effort and output is crucial.

The business world offers many success stories of entrepreneurs fulfilling their potential by pursuing and actualizing big dreams. We find particularly inspiring stories of new business ventures that do well—and do good. For example, Blake Mycoskie founded TOMS Shoes as part of the One for One Movement: For every pair of shoes the company sells, it donates a pair to a child in need in countries around the world. Mycoskie shares his vision and that of other "social entrepreneurs" in his book *Start Something That Matters.*[4]

To ignite school improvement requires *acting* on the belief that virtually all students (an estimated 95 percent, excepting only those with the most severe learning challenges) have the academic potential to develop critical reasoning and problem-solving abilities. Whole system education reform in Ontario, Canada, offers inspiring examples of the power of the UP Paradigm.[5] When administrators, teachers, and parents share in the belief that all children can learn when provided with effective instruction and opportunities to practice and develop their skills, they work together to actualize that belief through such improvements as embedded literacy coaches, principal leadership, professional development, budget allocations, parental involvement, and action research to identify what teaching and learning strategies are most effective. At one school in the York Region District near Toronto, elementary students' reading scores on a provincial test improved from 44 percent to 90 percent from third grade to sixth grade, writing went from 40 percent to 87 percent, and math improved from 50 percent to 83 percent as a result of those improvements.[6] In our work with the graduates of the master's and educational specialist degrees in brain-based teaching, we have seen that as educators develop a deeper belief in the untapped potential of their students and themselves, they set positive expectations and have high levels of motivation to teach students cognitive and metacognitive skills for becoming smarter adaptive learners.

Seven Principles of the Positively Smarter Approach

It is possible to make these examples the rule rather than the exception. In this book we have explored implications of research from a broad range of fields, from cognitive education, psychology, and educational neuroscience to exercise and nutrition science. We have also shared practical strategies for enhancing happiness and subjective well-being, achievement and productivity, and wellness and vitality. This exploration can be distilled into seven principles (see Figure 9.1).

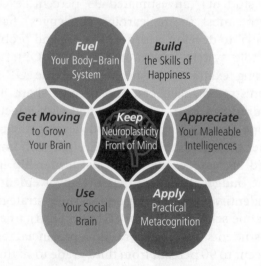

Figure 9.1 Seven Principles of Becoming Positively Smarter. © 2015 BrainSMART, Inc.

Principle 1: Keep Neuroplasticity Front of Mind

As you learn something new, challenge yourself to improve your skills, or practice strategies for enhancing optimism and happiness, you are in a sense reshaping your brain through the mechanism of neuroplasticity. The brain makes new neural connections and strengthens or weakens patterns of connections as a result of learning. You can take advantage of neuroplasticity throughout your life. Understanding this ability of your amazing brain can help motivate and inspire you to stay engaged in the work of becoming positively smarter over time.

Principle 2: Build the Skills of Optimism and Happiness

Your outlook is not an unchangeable trait, but a learnable, improvable skill. Honing your happiness and maintaining an optimistic attitude can have a significant impact on your performance and well-being. According to the *World Happiness Report*, the benefits of subjective well-being may include improved functioning of cardiovascular, immune, and endocrine systems; lower risk of heart disease and stroke; decreased susceptibility to infection; quicker recovery from illness; increased longevity; better work productivity; higher pay; enhanced creativity, problem solving, cooperation, and collaboration on the job; and more positive and fulfilling relationships.[7] A key strategy in maintaining a positive approach and improving your subjective well-being is to wield the CIA model to focus on factors that are within your control—that 40 percent of your outlook that is malleable. Instead of allowing your mind to wander into negative thoughts and worries, keep your selective attention on optimism. In this way, focus functions as the fulcrum of happiness.

Principle 3: Appreciate Your Potential to Become Smarter

Just as your outlook is malleable, so is your ability to develop your creative, practical, and analytical abilities—to become functionally smarter and to expand the knowledge and skills you need to achieve your personal and professional goals. In doing so, you can lead a more meaningful and purposeful life. By establishing your clear intent and setting ambitious, but achievable goals, you can make steady progress through the synergy of determination, well-paced effort, practice over time, and adherence to the motto of "progress over perfection." This synergy powers an upward spiral of greater achievement and happiness: Every step forward brings with it the motivating sense of accomplishment that inspires you to keep striving and enhances your belief in your ability to succeed.

Principle 4: Apply Practical Metacognition and Cognitive Assets

Practical metacognition—the process of establishing clear intent about what you want to achieve; planning and executing action steps; and assessing, monitoring, and adjusting your thoughts and actions so that you keep making progress—provides the framework for optimal use of your cognitive assets. Research indicates that cognitive skills can be learned, can be useful in all aspects of life, and can help you support a positive outlook. In this book, you learned about the cognitive assets of appropriate courage for tackling tough learning tasks, systematic search and planning, understanding and managing time, cognitive flexibility, learning from experience, and finishing power to complete tasks.

Principle 5: Use Your Social Brain to Enhance Well-Being and Achievement

There are many documented benefits for both mind and body from developing and maintaining positive social relationships. Social connections have been shown to support cardiovascular health, giving new meaning to the term *heart-healthy*; mental health, including a lessening of depression and anxiety; and brain health, in the form of slowing cognitive decline with aging. As with happiness and cognition, you can develop greater social skills across the life span by accentuating the positive; enhancing listening skills; considering others' points of view; learning together in partnership, within your social and professional circles and on the Internet; encouraging and supporting others; and participating actively in your various communities of family, friends, colleagues, neighbors, and organizations.

Principle 6: Get Moving to Grow Your Brain (and Become Fitter, Stronger, Smarter, and Happier)

Regular exercise has been shown to benefit people of all ages by starting young people on the right path and helping older adults to enjoy better health and sharper minds. Aerobic exercise and strength training support the creation of new neurons and synapses, increase angiogenesis, and are associated with brain areas involved in memory, spatial processing, and executive function. In studies of children, movement during the school day is associated with enhancing attention, supporting cognitive flexibility, and enhancing creativity. Smart strategies for increasing body-brain fitness include finding some form of exercise you enjoy; making exercise part of your routine; and putting the research into practice in your life.

Principle 7: Fuel Your Body–Brain System to Enhance Productivity and Learning

Like regular exercise, healthy nutrition habits can have a profoundly positive impact on ongoing happiness and help you achieve your goals and maintain well-being. The Mediterranean diet, rich in vegetables and fruits, beans and nuts, whole grains, fish, and olive oil, brings together heart- and brain-healthy nutrients. Practice healthy eating by using strategies such as eating more slowly and savoring meals while minimizing distractions; using small dishes and measuring portions and sharing when eating out; eating more vegetables, fruits, whole grains, and low-fat dairy for snacks and at mealtimes; and drinking plenty of water. Limit sugary and fatty foods and reduce sodium content.

Capitalize on Your Neurocognitive Synergy

As you begin to apply strategies for enhancing happiness, increasing achievement and productivity, exercising, and improving nutrition, you can achieve a synergistic effect on your Body–Brain System and your cognition and mood. Applying strategies to improve in any domain of becoming positively smarter—increasing your happiness, achievement, or well-being—can be extremely beneficial in its own right and have a positive, reinforcing impact in other areas as well. For example, through regular aerobic exercise and strength training, you can become fitter and stronger *and* improve your mood and subjective well-being. Regular exercise also helps to improve focus and attention to enhance achievement and supports neuroplasticity, neurogenesis, and angiogenesis in the brain. Exercise may support the creation of some 1,400 new neurons in the hippocampus each day, expanding your capacity to form new memories when learning new knowledge or skills.[8] Along the same lines, using strategies to influence the 40 percent of happiness that is most under your control can lead to smarter thinking in the achievement domain, better physical well-being, and benefits to the brain. By actively improving in one area, the synergistic spillover into all three domains can be substantial (see Figure 9.2).

The Practical Metacognition Process for Pursuing Important Goals

Now that we have summarized the research, theory, and strategies for improving happiness, achievement, and well-being, we move to a process for putting these ideas into practice. The practical metacognition approach, comprising clear intent, planning, execution, assessment, and ongoing progress, draws on evidence from the stages of change model set out by Carlo DiClemente and J. O. Prochaska in the 1980s. They define the stages as precontemplation, contemplation, determination, action, maintenance, and termination. A more recent version, by John Norcross in his work *Changeology*, found that matching the stages of change with

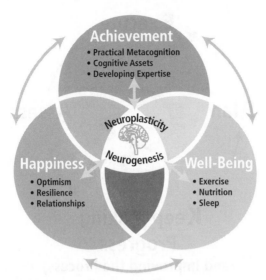

Figure 9.2 Components of Neurocognitive Synergy. © 2015 BrainSMART, Inc.

practical strategies makes a significant difference in the likelihood of achieving goals and changing behavior. In fact, more "action-oriented resolvers," those who moved from thinking about change to applying strategies, were 10 times more successful over six months than those who did not.[9] Applying practical metacognition to your goals of effecting positive changes in your life involves these steps, which we refer to as the PEAK process (see Figure 9.3):

1. **Establish your clear intent:** Formulate a positive, motivating goal, and envision the benefits the goal will bring.
2. **Plan:** Develop a specific plan for progressing in a positive direction. Focus on "when–then" planning to help to make your action steps more concrete. We are more likely to execute a plan when we specify exactly *when* we will do what we plan to do. For example: *When* I get up in the morning, *then* I will go for a run. *When* I go to a restaurant, *then* I will order salmon and a salad.

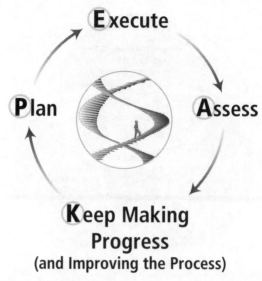

Figure 9.3 The PEAK Process for Optimizing Practical Metacognition. © 2015 BrainSMART, Inc.

3. **Execute:** Focus fully on executing action steps.
4. **Assess:** Assess, monitor, and adjust your thoughts and actions as you execute your plan and after you complete an action step.
5. **Keep making progress (and improving the process):** Aim for steady gains in a positive direction and be open to ways for improving the process.

Because it is a popular goal for an at-best-average, middle-aged athlete, Marcus offers this example of putting this process into practice in finishing a half-marathon, the fastest-growing distance event in the United States (the number of runners completing a half-marathon has quadrupled since 2000 to 1.96 million[10]).

Clear intent: To enjoy finishing a half-marathon. To trigger production of BDNF, which fuels neurogenesis and synaptogenesis as I learned new content (through our research for writing this book); as I got fitter, I also built more blood vessels (angiogenesis) in my Body–Brain System. To increase my creative capacities by generating new ideas for important projects and benefiting from the positive mood that flows from running.

Plan: *When* I first get up, *then* I will go for a run. I have my running gear ready to go, so there are no excuses for delay. I plan to run for 60 minutes at a heart rate of around 130 with a warm-up and cool-down period. My goal is to steadily build up over time.

Execute: I stuck to my plans for each step of the process; warmed up for 10 minutes; ran steadily with my heart rate around 130, and focused on my running form, cadence (steps per minute), and posture. At the end, I made sure I included a cool-down period.

Assess: I monitored and adjusted my thoughts and actions. For example, when my run went well in terms of heart rate, pace, and form, I started to think I should push it and run faster. I ignored the thoughts and kept the run steady. When I planned on a cadence of 180 but my heart rate rose because of heat, I slowed my pace. On my next run, I will focus more on cadence.

Keep making progress (and improving the process): I kept my focus on making steady progress over time and continued to improve my form.

This is a practical process that can applied to most goals. Note that the practical metacognition graphic (Figure 9.3) depicts a person climbing the steps of a spiral staircase. This is an apt visual metaphor for the steady process of taking progressively more difficult steps toward developing a skill.

Thanks for Joining Us on a Journey to Becoming Positively Smarter

Our goal in writing this book is to share with you some practical implications of educational neuroscience, current research about factors that can increase levels of happiness, achievement of important goals, development of skills that can make you functionally smarter, and ways in which exercise and nutrition can support your physical well-being. In addition, you can benefit from a positive synergy across these domains. We have also shared action assessments so you can see where you are currently and strategies for moving forward in any areas that are important to you.

As teacher educators, we have been sharing many of these concepts in live events and through graduate courses for almost 20 years. One of our greatest joys is to hear from people who have applied what we have shared and the positive results they have created. As we travel and present across the United States and internationally, it is exciting to meet graduates from the degree programs who share what they are doing to help to make their classrooms, schools, and organizations positively smarter. We look forward to hearing from you about how you are applying what you have learned in this book and the results you experience. We invite you to join us on www.InnovatingMinds.org for updates, events, and additional resources for helping you reach your goals. As the Scottish mountaineer W. H. Murray wrote: "Whatever you can do, or dream you can, begin it. Boldness has genius, power, and magic in it!"

Notes

1 Robert J. Sternberg. 1996. *Successful Intelligence: How Practical and Creative Intelligence Determine Success in Life.* New York: Putnam Penguin, p. 19.

2 Dan Millman. 2006. *Way of the Peaceful Warrior: A Book That Changes Lives* (rev. ed.). Tiburon, CA: HJ Kramer, p. 28.

3 Robert E. Kelley. 1998. *How to Be a Star at Work.* New York: Random House.

4 Blake Mycoskie. 2011. *Start Something That Matters.* New York: Spiegel & Grau.

5 Michael Fullan. 2010. *All Systems Go: The Change Imperative for Whole System Change.* Thousand Oaks, CA: Corwin Press.

6 Fullan, p. 45.

7 John Helliwell, Richard Layard, and Jeffrey Sachs, Editors. *World Happiness Report 2013.* New York: United Nations. Retrieved from http://unsdsn. org/wp-content/uploads/2014/02/WorldHappinessReport2013_online.pdf

8 William Skaggs. "New Neurons for New Memories: How Does the Brain Form New Memories Without Ever Filling Up?" *Scientific American Mind,* September/October 2014, pp. 49–53.

9 John C. Norcross. 2012. *Changeology: 5 Steps to Realizing Your Goals and Resolutions.* New York: Simon & Schuster, pp. 22–23.

10 Running USA. "Running USA's Annual, Half-Marathon Report," April 16, 2014. Retrieved from http://www.runningusa.org/index.cfm?fuseaction= news.details&ArticleId=333

Appendix: Positively Smarter Action Assessment

1. Focus on a Positive Outlook

On a daily basis, how often do you . . .	Almost never	Sometimes	Frequently	Consistently
1. Savor the wow of now.				
2. Work at consciously maintaining an upbeat attitude.				
3. Picture a positive future.				
4. Actively commit acts of kindness.				
5. Acknowledge and appreciate the good things in your life.				

(continued)

1. Focus on a Positive Outlook (*cont'd*)

On a daily basis, how often do you …	Almost never	Sometimes	Frequently	Consistently
6. Recognize and set aside negative thoughts and worries.				
7. Take time to relate to others in positive ways.				
8. Achieve a state of flow or find yourself "in the zone."				
9. Set and monitor your progress toward positive goals.				
10. Respond with resilience to tough challenges.				
11. Look past others' real and imagined transgressions to let go of anger and resentment.				
12. Move your body to boost your mood.				
13. Smile frequently and naturally.				
14. Play to your peak strength.				
15. Identify and share the treasures in your life.				

2. Work Toward Your Goals

On a daily basis, how often do you . . .	*Almost never*	*Sometimes*	*Frequently*	*Consistently*
1. Move outside your comfort zone to take positive risks.				
2. Set your sights on mastering new skills and knowledge rather than relying on external performance measures.				
3. Identify and build on your strengths.				
4. Establish step-by-step objectives to work toward achieving larger goals.				
5. Pace yourself to head off burnout.				
6. Aim for progress, not perfection.				
7. Picture your success to maintain focus, motivation, and momentum.				
8. Employ effective strategies to improve retention of important information.				

3. Employ Cognitive Assets to Work Smarter

On a daily basis, how often do you ...	Almost never	Sometimes	Frequently	Consistently
1. Establish your clear intent.				
2. Proceed with appropriate courage through the steps you need to accomplish your goals.				
3. Engage in systematic planning and searches for the information you need to work smarter.				
4. Manage your time wisely.				
5. Accurately assess situations and adjust your thoughts and actions accordingly.				
6. Learn from experience.				
7. Finish what you start.				

4. Hone Your Social Intelligence

On a daily basis, how often do you ...	Almost never	Sometimes	Frequently	Consistently
1. Accentuate the positive in your interactions with others.				
2. Listen effectively.				
3. Carefully consider others' points of view.				
4. Consciously establish rapport.				
5. Take advantage of opportunities to learn with others.				
6. Encourage and support others.				
7. Participate actively in and contribute to your many "communities."				

5. Work Out Your Body–Brain System

In a typical week, how often do you . . .	*1–3 times*	*4–6 times*	*Daily*	*Total time (in minutes)*
1. Engage in aerobic exercise that raises your heart and respiratory rate.				
2. Engage in strength training that works out all your major muscle groups.				

6. Choose Healthy Foods for Your Body–Brain System

In your daily diet, do you ...	Almost never	Sometimes	Frequently	Consistently
1. Make fruits and vegetables part of meals and snacks (nine servings a day, excluding potatoes).				
2. Choose lean protein.				
3. Understand the role of omega-3 fatty acids in maintaining heart and brain health and incorporate these good fats into your diet.				
4. Choose whole grains over refined flours.				
5. Minimize your intake of trans fats, saturated fats, sugar, and sodium.				
6. Pay attention to portion size.				
7. Set positive goals for healthy eating.				

Index

Page locators in *italic* type indicate figures.

Positively Smarter: Science and Strategies for Increasing Happiness, Achievement, and Well-Being,
First Edition. Marcus Conyers and Donna Wilson.
© 2015 John Wiley & Sons, Inc. Published 2015 by John Wiley & Sons, Inc.

About the Authors

Marcus Conyers is the author and coauthor of 20 books, book chapters, and articles on cultivating creative and critical thinking skills, developing expert performance, and maintaining a healthy Body–Brain System. Marcus serves as director of communications for the Center for Innovative Education and Prevention. He has worked in 30 countries and is an international keynote speaker whose audiences have included ministers of education in South Africa, the United Arab Emirates, and Ontario, Canada. He has presented at academic conferences at universities in the United States and Canada, at the University of Cambridge in the United Kingdom, and at Leiden University in the Netherlands. Marcus has worked with a broad range of groups in education, business, counter-intelligence, counter-terrorism, special forces, law enforcement, and fire and rescue. With his passion for fitness, he runs half-marathons in the United States and rows in the Cambridge Town Bumps in England.

Donna Wilson, PhD, is an educational/school psychologist and teacher educator who completed post-doctoral studies in structural cognitive modifiability. She is former chair of education at

Positively Smarter: Science and Strategies for Increasing Happiness, Achievement, and Well-Being, First Edition. Marcus Conyers and Donna Wilson.
© 2015 John Wiley & Sons, Inc. Published 2015 by John Wiley & Sons, Inc.

the University of Detroit Mercy and a current adjunct professor at Nova Southeastern University. Donna has led on district, community, and state initiatives that have put some key concepts from this book into practice, and she presents at US policy conferences to help bridge the gap between research and practice in education. She is the author and coauthor of more than 30 professional books, book chapters, and articles and is an active contributor to the online educational community.

Together, Donna and Marcus codeveloped master's and educational specialist degrees with majors in brain-based teaching and a doctoral minor in brain-based leadership with the Abraham S. Fischler School of Education at Nova Southeastern University. These programs are among the first in this emerging field, also known as educational neuroscience/mind, brain and education, which melds research from fields including cognitive psychology, education, and neuroscience. Today, graduates from 47 states and 12 countries are applying what they learned in these programs. Donna and Marcus are the authors of *Five Big Ideas for Effective Teaching: Connecting Mind, Brain, and Education Research to Classroom Practice.*